Survivorship
Living Well During and After Cancer

Barrie Cassileth, PhD
Memorial Sloan-Kettering Cancer Center

with Ian Yarett

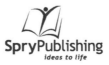

SpryPublishing
ideas to life

This edition is published by Spry Publishing LLC
2500 South State Street
Ann Arbor, MI 48104 USA

Printed and bound in the United States of America.

10 9 8 7 6 5 4 3 2 1

Library of Congress Control Number: 2013949027

Paperback ISBN: 978-1-938170-35-5
E-book ISBN: 978-1-938170-36-2

Disclaimer: Spry Publishing LLC does not assume responsibility
for the contents or opinions expressed herein. Although every precaution
is taken to ensure that information is accurate as of the date of
publication, differences of opinion exist. The opinions expressed herein
are those of the author and do not necessarily reflect the views of the
publisher. The information contained in this book is not intended to
replace professional advisement of an individual's doctor prior to
beginning or changing an individual's course of treatment.

To my husband and children
for their forebearance, support, and creative ideas,
with all my love and appreciation.

To our patients
for their remarkable bravery and our
integrative therapists and physicians for
their devotion and expertise.

To patients and cancer therapists everywhere
for their ability to give and live to the fullest under
the most difficult of circumstances.

A special thanks
to Ian Yarett. We were fortunate to have him
with us at MSKCC for a year before he started
medical school, and he worked tirelessly to
put together the first draft of this book.

Contents

Preface

Many years ago, I completed a doctorate in medical sociology at the University of Pennsylvania. For my thesis project, I chose to spend a year studying the dynamics of care on the adult leukemia unit of the Penn's Cancer Center, a small cluster of beds adjacent to the Center's research laboratories. What I found that year not only became my thesis, it molded my lifelong profession.

I found a world filled with terribly ill adults, mostly young or in their middle years, and I encountered their husbands, wives, parents, and children, all of whom suffered just as much, knowing that the prolonged and difficult treatments had a small chance of success. Physicians, nurses, and other staff faced similar challenges as they guided their patients through treatment, aware of its limitations and of the gaps in scientific knowledge underlying it.

It became clear to me that more was needed than simply caring for each patient's leukemia, as difficult and consuming as that was. A host of physical, emotional, and interpersonal problems screamed for attention. Identifying them and outlining ways to approach them became my thesis and later a book, *The Cancer Patient: Social and Medical Aspects of Care*.

After that year, I was asked to stay on to establish a program that could address these issues. We called it the "Psychosocial Program." Under that rubric we created support services for patients, families, and staff, established the first palliative care and home hospice programs based in an academic medical center, and conducted multiple research studies.

In 1999, I was invited to bring all that I had learned and developed over the previous decades to Memorial Sloan-Kettering Cancer Center, the world's preeminent cancer hospital, and to create a new kind of department, an Integrative Medicine department. This was an opportunity not only to bring the field to a new plateau, but to produce a program that could be a prototype for other hospitals around the world, and that is exactly what happened. The various elements of our program focus on patients' needs throughout the full spectrum of their treatment and well beyond. Helping survivors and their loved ones to live strong and stay well is the major goal of what we do. Survivorship from diagnosis on presents new challenges, and survivorship is what this book is about.

— Barrie Cassileth

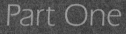

Part One

Information to Start

A Roadmap
for Quality Care

Despite the statistics, we tend to believe that cancer happens to other people—those who are older or sicker or have less healthy habits—but not to us. Invariably, it's not something for which we are prepared. A diagnosis of cancer changes everything. It makes us unsure when once we were certain, and the unfairness and scariness of it all hit us and our loved ones hard.

Questions, from the profound to the practical, swirl in our heads: Why me? Could I have done something to prevent this? Is it treatable or curable? Can it be removed through surgery? What side effects will result from any surgery or other treatments? What on earth can I do, should I do, and how will this diagnosis and its treatment affect my life and my family?

This book is designed to help you navigate your options, make informed choices, and maintain the highest quality of life possible during and after this challenging time.

Some General Guidelines for Facing Your Cancer

No matter how resilient a person you are, an unexpected and frightening diagnosis brings about a great deal of uncertainty. It's entirely normal to feel overwhelmed, anxious, or even angry. Many cancer patients experience a feeling of losing control over their lives and the sense that their autonomy is taking a backseat to the disease. Addressing your physical disease in a way that also allows you to confront the roller coaster of emotions that comes along with it is not only possible, but also essential to your overall well-being and that of your family.

Anxiety and uncertainty are reduced when people take an active role in their own treatment, and often this also leads to getting the best quality care. When facing cancer, it is true that some elements that may contribute to the final outcome are beyond control, but you can benefit tremendously by taking charge of those choices you do have. You can decide which doctors and hospitals to use. You can take an active and informed role as a partner in decisions about your treatment plan. You can choose to make lifestyle changes such as diet and exercise, which improve health and well-being and even survival.

Additionally, you can take advantage of various complementary (integrative) therapies that reduce physical and emotional symptoms along the way. Don't allow the unfortunate challenges of cancer to run the show. With conscious effort you can remain in the driver's seat of your future. In this book, we will show you how.

Take Charge! Here's What You Can Do
- Select the best doctor and hospital for your exact diagnosis.
- Take an active role in discussions and decisions about your treatment plan.
- Never hesitate to ask questions of your oncology team.
- Make lifestyle changes that improve well-being and survival.
- Use complementary (integrative) therapies as adjuncts to mainstream care to control physical and emotional symptoms.

The remainder of this chapter provides a roadmap for getting the best possible treatment and introduces the promise of complementary medicine and the potential perils of unproven "alternative" methods. Being an educated consumer will help you get the best treatment, and it also will improve both your outlook and how you feel each day.

Your First Steps for Getting Quality Care

There is a critical decision to be made as soon as you receive a questionable test result or perhaps even a tentative cancer diagnosis. Where do you go to confirm the specific diagnosis and receive medical care? Where you are diagnosed and treated first can have a major impact on the ultimate outcome, so it is very important to start at a specialized cancer center that sees many patients with your specific condition. Your initial leaning may be to use your community hospital where you feel comfortable, but with a cancer diagnosis, that might not be the best first-step choice. Specialized cancer centers have oncologists with the most expertise and experience in diagnosing and treating your specific problem.

If you prefer, when diagnosis and treatment plans are established and initial treatment requiring highly specialized physicians and facilities is completed, you can then take your continuing treatment plan to your local hospital for any ongoing treatments. In cancer treatment, excellence and specialization are keys to success.

Cancer Centers

While most, if not all, hospitals provide cancer treatment, specialized cancer centers offer the most highly developed professional care. The National Cancer Act of 1971 designated "cancer centers" as institutions that include excellence in patient care, training and education, research, high-level technologies, and cancer-control research and programs. According to the National Cancer Institute (NCI) website, the model for a cancer center was drawn from the older, free-standing institutions, including Roswell Park, Memorial Sloan-Kettering, M.D. Anderson, and Fox Chase.

In June 1973, the NCI described two classes of cancer centers—"comprehensive" and "specialized." Comprehensive cancer centers conduct long-term, multidisciplinary cancer programs in biomedical research, clinical investigation, training, demonstration, and community-oriented programs in detection, diagnosis, education, epidemiology, rehabilitation, and information exchange. Specialized cancer centers have programs in one or more, but not all, of the above areas.

Thus, NCI-designated comprehensive cancer centers are top of the line, having demonstrated depth and breadth of research, professional and public education, dissemination of clinical and public health advances, and, most importantly, the most knowledgeable cancer-diagnosis-specific, highest-quality patient care.

Included is a list of all 41 NCI-designated comprehensive cancer centers as of this writing, organized by state.

UAB Comprehensive Cancer Center, University of Alabama at Birmingham Birmingham, Alabama
(205) 975-8222 www3.ccc.uab.edu

University of Arizona Cancer Center, Tucson, Arizona
(520) 694-CURE (2873) azcc.arizona.edu

Chao Family Comprehensive Cancer Center, University of California, Irvine Orange, California
(714) 456-8600 www.cancer.uci.edu

City of Hope Comprehensive Cancer Center
Duarte, California
(626) 256-HOPE (4673) www.cityofhope.org/

Jonsson Comprehensive Cancer Center, University of California at Los Angeles Los Angeles, California
(888) 662-8252 www.cancer.ucla.edu

Moores Cancer Center, University of California, San Diego
La Jolla, California
(858) 657-7000 cancer.ucsd.edu

UC Davis Comprehensive Cancer Center, University of California at Davis Sacramento, California
(916) 734-5959 www.ucdmc.ucdavis.edu/cancer

UCSF Helen Diller Family Comprehensive Cancer Center, University of California at San Francisco San Francisco, California
(888) 689-8273 cancer.ucsf.edu

USC Norris Comprehensive Cancer Center, University of Southern California Los Angeles, California
(323) 865-3000 uscnorriscancer.usc.edu

University of Colorado Cancer Center
Aurora, Colorado
(303) 724-3155 www.uch.edu/colorado-cancer-center

Yale Cancer Center, Yale University School of Medicine
New Haven, Connecticut
(203) 785-4095 yalecancercenter.org

Georgetown Lombardi Comprehensive Cancer Center
Washington, DC
(202) 444-4000   lombardi.georgetown.edu

Moffitt Cancer Center
Tampa, Florida
(888) 663-3488   www.moffitt.org

Robert H. Lurie Comprehensive Cancer Center of Northwestern University   Chicago, Illinois
(312) 695-0990   cancer.northwestern.edu

University of Chicago Medicine Comprehensive Cancer Center
Chicago, Illinois
(773) 702-6180   cancer.uchicago.edu

Holden Comprehensive Cancer Center, The University of Iowa
Iowa City, Iowa
(319) 356-4200   www.uihealthcare.org/holdencomprehensivecancercenter

Sidney Kimmel Comprehensive Cancer Center, Johns Hopkins University   Baltimore, Maryland
(410) 955-5222   www.hopkinsmedicine.org/kimmel_cancer_center

Dana-Farber/Harvard Cancer Center
Boston, Massachusetts
(617) 632-3000   www.dfhcc.harvard.edu

Barbara Ann Karmanos Cancer Institute, Wayne State University School of Medicine   Detroit, Michigan
(800) 527-6266   www.karmanos.org

University of Michigan Comprehensive Cancer Center
Ann Arbor, Michigan
(734) 936-1831   mcancer.org

Masonic Cancer Center, University of Minnesota
Minneapolis, Minnesota
(612) 625-5411   cancer.umn.edu

Mayo Clinic Cancer Center   Rochester, Minnesota
(507) 284-2511   www.mayoclinic.org/mayo-clinic-cancer-center

Alvin J. Siteman Cancer Center, Washington University School of Medicine and Barnes-Jewish Hospital St. Louis, Missouri
(314) 747-3046 www.siteman.wustl.edu

Norris Cotton Cancer Center, Dartmouth-Hitchcock Medical Center
Lebanon, New Hampshire
(603) 653-9000 cancer.dartmouth.edu

Cancer Institute of New Jersey/Rutgers University
New Brunswick, New Jersey
(732) 235-2465 www.cinj.org

Herbert Irving Comprehensive Cancer Center, Columbia University
New York, New York
(212) 851-4680 hiccc.columbia.edu

Memorial Sloan-Kettering Cancer Center New York, New York
(212) 639-2000 www.mskcc.org

Roswell Park Cancer Institute Buffalo, New York
(716) 845-2300 www.roswellpark.org

Duke Cancer Institute, Duke University Medical Center
Durham, North Carolina
(888) 275-3853 www.dukecancerinstitute.org

UNC Lineberger Comprehensive Cancer Center, N.C. Cancer Hospital
Chapel Hill, North Carolina
(919) 966-3036 www.nccancerhospital.org

The Comprehensive Cancer Center of Wake Forest University
Winston-Salem, North Carolina
(888) 716-9253 www.wakehealth.edu/Comprehensive-Cancer-Center

Case Comprehensive Cancer Center, Case Western Reserve University
Cleveland, Ohio
(216) 844-8797 cancer.case.edu

Comprehensive Cancer Center–James Cancer Hospital and Solove Research Institute, The Ohio State University Columbus, Ohio
(614) 293-5066 cancer.osu.edu

Abramson Cancer Center, University of Pennsylvania
Philadelphia, Pennsylvania
(800) 789-7366 www.penncancer.org

Fox Chase Cancer Center Philadelphia, Pennsylvania
(888) 369-2427 www.fccc.edu

University of Pittsburgh Cancer Institute Pittsburgh, Pennsylvania
(412) 647-2811 www.upci.upmc.edu

St. Jude Children's Research Hospital Memphis, Tennessee
(901) 595-3300 www.stjude.org

Vanderbilt-Ingram Cancer Center, Vanderbilt University
Nashville, Tennessee
(877) 936-8422 www.vicc.org

M.D. Anderson Cancer Center, University of Texas Houston, Texas
(713) 792-2121 www.mdanderson.org

**Fred Hutchinson/University of Washington Cancer Consortium,
Fred Hutchinson Cancer Research Center** Seattle, Washington
(206) 667-5000 fhcrc.org

UW Carbone Comprehensive Cancer Center, University of Wisconsin
Madison, Wisconsin
(800) 622-8922 www.uwhealth.org/cancer

Advice at the Outset

First, the best advice is to find the nearest NCI-designated comprehensive cancer center. Because there are 41 of these centers across the country, no matter where you live at least one should be within a few hours' drive of your home. Most of these specialty cancer hospitals are affiliated with major academic medical centers and are leaders in cancer research and pioneers of the latest and best cancer treatments. You can ask your primary care physician to refer you to a specialist at an NCI-designated comprehensive cancer center, or you can call yourself and make an appointment to see one of the top specialists in your specific type of cancer.

Even if you prefer to receive treatment at a local hospital closer to home, it is still important to get this high-level initial consultation to confirm your exact diagnosis and clinical status and to get a specific treatment plan. Specialists at comprehensive cancer centers have the experience to confirm your diagnosis specifically and to ensure that it is accurate and complete. They can then prescribe an appropriate treatment plan based on the latest scientific evidence.

If surgery or other needed treatment is especially complex, you may prefer to have it at the comprehensive center with a team that specializes in your particular type and location of disease. Some advanced diagnostic and treatment facilities are available only at the major cancer centers. When you have a confirmed diagnosis and a treatment plan, you can decide to complete the treatment at the comprehensive cancer center or return home with your treatment prescription to receive your treatment locally. Your local oncologist will always be able to contact and correspond with his or her counterpart at the comprehensive center. If need be, you can always return to the comprehensive center for follow-up consultation tests and advice as needed.

Serious potential problems will be avoided by seeing experts at a comprehensive center right after a tentative diagnosis. It will avoid such worst-case scenarios as receiving an incorrect or insufficient diagnosis or suboptimal treatment, avoiding time delays when time is of the essence.

What about Complementary and "Alternative" Medicine?

The good news is that, thanks to the latest medical advances, millions of cancer patients—the great majority—live for many years after being diagnosed. But the conventional, evidence-based care delivered by oncologists that has made this possible is sometimes lacking in other aspects of care. While conventional care in the hospital setting can be extraordinarily successful at treating the tumor, it can also feel very impersonal. Cancer patients' physical and emotional symptoms may fall through the cracks. Where conventional therapies such as chemotherapy and radiation treat the tumor, adjunctive *complementary* (integrative) therapies treat physical and emotional symptoms. At least some adjunctive complementary therapies are available in virtually all major cancer centers, as well as in many community hospitals.

Cynthia, age 36 with advanced-stage gynecologic cancer, commenting on massage therapy

"Knowing I can count on a massage and on this kind of bodywork has made a huge difference. It's hard to describe what being touched is like during this time, but everything has been so frightening—the diagnosis, the chemo, the pain, the side effects. I am so unbelievably anxious—and your touch helps me so much."

Complementary therapies do not treat the cancer itself. Instead, they effectively control physical and emotional symptoms and promote general health and well-being. Such therapies include meditation, self-hypnosis, yoga, acupuncture treatment, music therapy, massage therapy, healthy diets, exercise, and more. It is worth repeating that complementary therapies should never be used *instead of* conventional cancer care. Rather, they are important adjuncts to use along with proper cancer care. Many highly promoted remedies are falsely touted to cancer patients as "miracle cures," but the old adage about sounding too good to be true applies here. (We'll discuss this much more in the next section.)

Unfortunately, dissatisfied with the treatment options available to them and looking to take control of their own health and healing, some cancer patients turn instead to a variety of unconventional therapists for "alternative cancer treatments." These include naturopathy, ayurveda, herbalism, homeopathy, special diets, expensive bogus approaches such as oxygen therapy, bioelectromagnetism, and numerous others.

> No "alternative" treatments have been shown through research to cure or treat cancer.

It is important to realize that no "alternative" treatments have been shown through research to cure or treat cancer, despite promoter claims to the contrary. These bogus "alternative" treatments must be separated from complementary therapies, which are evidence based and used to control symptoms and enhance well-being. Respected complementary therapies are detailed in parts 2 and 3.

Our goal in this book is to provide you with clear, objective, and easy-to-use information and resources to help you take advantage of the most useful and scientifically validated complementary modalities, while avoiding those that are unproven or potentially harmful. Information—including much misinformation—abounds on these topics. We hope this book will help light the way as you explore your options.

What Integrative Medicine Is … and Isn't

Integrative medicine takes advantage of complementary therapies such as acupuncture, massage, meditation, guided imagery and self-hypnosis, and yoga. The field especially emphasizes the crucial importance of good nutrition and physical activity. Always along with, not instead of conventional cancer care, integrative medicine incorporates these and other modalities to manage symptoms that may occur during and remain after completion of cancer treatment. Integrative therapies reduce both short- and long-term side effects, such as pain and anxiety. They can relieve stress, promote general well-being, and, in some cases, reduce the risk of cancer recurrence.

According to the Consortium of Academic Health Centers for Integrative Medicine, there are yet other integrative medicine benefits: it "reaffirms the importance of the relationship between practitioner and patient, focuses on the whole person, is informed by evidence, and makes use of all appropriate therapeutic approaches, healthcare professionals, and disciplines to achieve optimal health and healing."

> ### Jimmy, 45-years old, under treatment for diffuse large B-cell lymphoma
>
> "This hasn't been the easiest time, but one thing I've really appreciated about having to be in the hospital was the acupuncture, massage, music, and mind-body sessions. They've really helped this all be less awful."

The Important Difference between Complementary and Alternative Medicine

In the realm of integrative medicine or integrative oncology, terminology can be very confusing. "Complementary" and "alternative" are sometimes used synonymously, and the acronym "CAM" (complementary and alternative medicine) perpetuates the problem. However, here is a better set of terms used by integrative medicine specialists and increasingly by others: "Alternative medicine" is understood to mean treatments promoted for use *instead of* conventional cancer therapy. "Complementary therapies" are treatments used *in conjunction with* conventional care.

"Alternative" medicine encompasses a broad array of unconventional treatment modalities that are generally either unproven or were disproved in scientific studies. Examples are listed in the appendix at the end of the book. "Complementary" therapies, on the other hand, are rational and scientifically validated for symptom control use along with mainstream cancer care.

Some modalities that have an appropriate complementary

usage may be considered by some for use in *treating* cancer instead, making that use "alternative" instead of complementary. An example is the use of acupuncture for symptom control (a very helpful complementary therapy), but use of acupuncture to *treat* cancer would be a useless "alternative" treatment as illustrated in the Steve Jobs cautionary tale that follows. Alternative techniques are to be avoided. They can be dangerous as well as useless.

Acupuncture, massage therapy, and music therapy, among other modalities, have been shown to be safe and effective as complementary treatments for managing pain, nausea, stress, and many other symptoms, and for supporting overall patient well-being. Their growing use in mainstream cancer settings is known as "integrative oncology."

Important Distinction

Be wary of any claim that a non-mainstream technique (something other than surgery, chemotherapy, radiation therapy, etc.) can treat or cure cancer. Be wary even when such approaches use the term "integrative." Whether such claims are products of wishful thinking or malicious scams, they are not supported by scientific research. Second, remember that complementary (also called integrative) therapies, by definition, must be used in conjunction with or following the conclusion of, not instead of, conventional care. Complementary therapies, helpful as they can be, are not in themselves curative. However, when used along with mainstream care, they can help you weather both the disease and any negative side effects of cancer and its treatments as well.

Steve Jobs—A Cautionary Tale

The story of Steve Jobs' battle with pancreatic cancer, as told by his biographer Walter Issacson, provides a cautionary tale in the use of "alternative" medicine. Employees and friends of the iconic Apple CEO joked that he generated a "reality-distortion field," allowing him to make up rules as he went along and to create products and even whole new product categories without any prior evidence that people would want them. Many would argue that this was Jobs' unique brand of brilliance, and few would deny that it served him well in business. But unfortunately, when it comes to cancer or any similar disease, wishful thinking isn't enough.

Jobs was diagnosed with pancreatic cancer in 2003 after a CT scan to look for kidney stones showed a "shadow" on his pancreas. Although pancreatic cancer is one of the most deadly malignancies, Jobs' particular type (a neuroendocrine islet tumor) was slow growing and treatable, with a relatively good prognosis. Nevertheless, he opted not to have surgery and sought to treat his disease through diet and other alternative means. He eventually agreed to the surgery nine months later when doctors found that the cancer had spread. Jobs underwent a liver transplant and sought out experimental treatments, but ultimately died on Oct. 5, 2011, at age 56.

Of course, we cannot know for sure what would have been. Perhaps, despite the favorable odds, mainstream treatment may not have been able to save him or extend his life. But turning to surgery earlier and using complementary medicine as an adjunct to, rather than a replacement for, conventional care likely would have given him a better chance.

In the absence of certainty about the best way forward, following the medical evidence—albeit incomplete and constantly evolving—is usually the safest option. Also remember that preventing disease is not the same as curing it. Eating well, exercising regularly, and so on can indeed help decrease the risk of cancer and other diseases, but they can't be expected to cure disease on their own.

Knowledge Is Power, but Consider the Source

An enormous amount of information about integrative medicine can be found in printed sources and online. But again, a word of caution—some of this information is high quality and scientifically validated, and some is not. Some is downright ugly, as there are many scam artists out there promoting bogus remedies and cures.

At present, a simple Google search for "alternative cancer" produces close to 62 million hits! Two examples of sites that rank highly in that search and should be avoided—Cancer-Tutor.com and Alternative-Cancer.net—are representative examples of the numerous sites that provide and/or sell "advice" on a range of therapies purported to cure cancer without mainstream treatment. On the other hand, there are useful sites that debunk false information, such as QuackWatch.org, and others that provide good information on complementary treatments, their risks, and their benefits. (A list of reliable information sources can be found in the resources section at the end of the book.)

The problem of quackery has been recorded since the seventeenth century. Some quacks are true charlatans with purely financial motives, while others are believers in what they preach. Both, however, promote unproven or disproved alternative therapies as cures for disease. And, unfortunately, there is no shortage of patients willing to embark on these questionable and often very expensive treatment plans. Desperate patients and their loved ones are inclined to believe

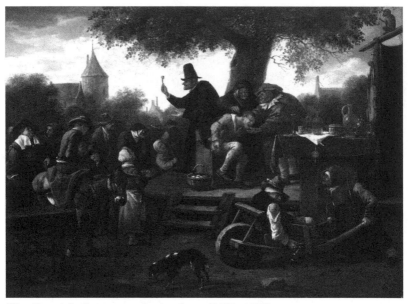

"The Quack," oil on canvas by Jan Steen (1626–1679).

in miracles—particularly when facing serious or untreatable illnesses.

The truth is that unproven approaches are dangerous to patients. Even when the therapy itself does not harm, people too often choose to shun conventional treatment entirely and replace it with an alternative treatment that does nothing to diminish their disease. Public education can help, along with knowledgeable doctors who are familiar enough with alternative approaches to successfully guide patients away from them.

In the remaining chapters of this book, we will focus on complementary therapies, designed to be used in conjunction with mainstream cancer treatment. When used correctly, these therapies can provide relief, both during treatment and following treatment, of side effects caused by cancer treatments or by the cancer itself.

Part Two

Complementary Therapies—The Basics

Benjamin, age 54 with leukemia, discussing outpatient massage therapy

"I felt like you came for 'me,' and not for my disease, which is why everyone else comes, too. You helped 'the whole me,' not just the cancer, and I've learned so much about how to relax, and breathe, and calm down. Thank you so much."

What Complementary Therapies Can Do for You

Complementary therapies empower you, the patient. After being diagnosed with cancer, you might feel like you are ceding control to a team of experts—your medical oncologist, radiation oncologist, and surgeon, not to mention their nurses and technicians. Together, all of these experts can give you the best quality care available for your condition. But it's not uncommon to feel lost in such a system.

Integrative medicine puts the ball back in your court. It

offers a broad array of therapies and lifestyle choices that not only make a real difference for your health and happiness, but also give you back a sense and reality of control and confidence.

There are many things you can do to maintain the best possible physical and emotional health throughout your cancer treatment and beyond. You can eat better, be physically active, and manage your stress through mind-body techniques. Acupuncture treatment and massage therapy will help minimize unwanted symptoms of chemotherapy or radiation. For example, studies suggest that acupuncture can be very helpful for reducing nausea and vomiting, as well as hot flashes that may arise if you are prescribed hormonal therapy. Acupuncture is successful at promoting relaxation, reducing stress, and diminishing pain, as well.

Most major cancer centers across the country, and many community hospitals, now have integrative medicine departments that offer some or all of these therapies, both on an in-patient and outpatient basis. Talk to your oncologist, but also consider speaking with a physician who specializes in integrative medicine or an expert in integrative medicine who specializes in working with cancer patients. They can help guide you to the best complementary therapies for particular problems. They can help you develop a comprehensive treatment plan that achieves the greatest synergy between the mainstream and complementary domains, giving you the best chance of beating your cancer while helping you live as comfortably as possible through the course of treatment and thereafter.

Modalities in the integrative medicine realm can be categorized in different ways. Some involve long-term lifestyle changes, and others are treatments you can receive from a practitioner once a week or so. Still others you can learn and then practice entirely on your own in the comfort of your own home.

Before we begin a discussion of specific complementary therapies, it is important to consider how researchers determine if a particular therapy works, or doesn't. It is research results that provide confidence that a therapy may provide the desired result.

What Is Proper Research?

In proper research, following promising clinical or laboratory results, a new therapy is pilot tested to determine best dosage and other important preliminary information. If the new therapy appears safe and effective, a larger, more definitive clinical trial is conducted. This trial will be "randomized," which means that patients will be randomly assigned to receive or not receive the therapy during the trial's duration. Determined by an electronic version of a coin-toss random allocation, patients will either belong to a group receiving the new treatment or to a group receiving the standard treatment for that specific cancer diagnosis.

Then, the two or more groups of subjects are followed in exactly the same way, receiving the same tests, visits, etc. Patients and their caregivers do not know to which group they were randomly assigned. Proper randomization balances known and unknown factors that might influence results, helping to assure that their results are not influenced by patient perceptions and are valid. Randomized clinical trials are lengthy and expensive, but they have produced the major advances in cancer treatment that led to the more than 67 percent survival rate of U.S. patients across all cancers.

Complementary treatments offer cancer patients many important advantages. They range from extended survival (exercise) to relieving stress, anxiety, and other symptoms (acupuncture, mind-body therapies, etc.). The several types of complementary therapies that have been studied and found to be beneficial for many cancer patients are profiled on the pages that follow, along with warnings as needed. Beneficial approaches include: diet and being savvy about supplements, physical fitness, acupuncture, mind-body therapies, massage therapies, and creative therapies. In the sections that follow, we'll look at each of these beneficial approaches, the research results, and what benefit each may offer to cancer patients.

Mary, 47-years old with multiple myeloma

"I was so surprised that guided imagery really helped me. I almost felt childish at first, like escaping to a fantasy world, but really enjoying the visualization actually allowed me to feel free and powerful. I don't have to be trapped by my circumstances; I can choose how to help myself through this."

Diet and Supplements

What you eat matters. A simple, perhaps obvious fact, but one that is too frequently overlooked. There is little doubt that what we eat has an impact on our risk of diseases such as cancer, and on the progression of those diseases after diagnosis. The nature of this connection has been, and continues to be, the subject of much scientific research. Although we have a lot more to learn, certain guidelines are becoming well established.

Excessive consumption of red meat, highly processed meats, and other sources of animal fat seems to promote cancer, whereas increased consumption of fruits, vegetables, whole grains, and low-fat animal foods may help to hinder it. Some important basic principles follow. A prospective study of 4,577 men with prostate cancer found that eating foods with trans fat, also called unsaturated fat, was associated with increased risk of all-cause death. Replacing carbohydrates and animal fat with vegetable fat may reduce the risk of all-cause death in prostate cancer, and consumption of vegetable fat may benefit men with prostate cancer.[1]

In a major overview of large, high-quality studies in patients with breast cancer, most found that higher intake of saturated fat before diagnosis was associated with increased risk of death. Moreover, higher monounsaturated fat intake both before and after breast cancer diagnosis was associated with increased risk of cancer-specific and all-cause mortality. Although further research is needed, it appears that consumption of "bad" fats increases breast cancer recurrence and mortality, whereas omega-3 fats seem to be beneficial.[2]

The bottom line is that lifestyle choices matter for improving survival after a cancer diagnosis. Survivors should continue to focus on maintaining a healthy weight, being physically active, avoiding smoking, and choosing a diet comprised of fruits and vegetables, lean protein, whole grains, and low-fat foods, including dairy. Replacing carbohydrates and animal fat with vegetables is a smart move. It improves survival in patients with cancer.[3]

Being diagnosed with cancer brings up many questions. Should I change my diet? Should I gain or lose weight? What diet will help me lose weight? Would I benefit from taking a multivitamin or other dietary supplements? Do healing diets work, and if so, which is best? You may also have heard inconsistent or confusing answers to these kinds of questions.

Dietary Fats

As outlined on the Mayo Clinic website,[4] there are two main types of harmful dietary fat: saturated fat and trans fats. These are solid at room temperature and include beef fat, pork fat, shortening, stick margarine, and butter.

Saturated fat. This comes mainly from animal sources of food. Saturated fat raises total blood cholesterol levels and low-density lipoprotein (LDL) cholesterol levels, which increase your risk of disease and could impact survival after cancer.

Trans fat. This occurs naturally in some foods, especially foods from animals. But most trans fats are made during food processing through partial hydrogenation of unsaturated fats, which creates fats that are easier to cook with and less likely to spoil than are natural oils. However, that can increase unhealthy LDL cholesterol and decrease healthy high-density lipoprotein (HDL) cholesterol, increasing the risk of disease.

Healthier dietary foods contain mostly monounsaturated and polyunsaturated fats. They are liquid at room temperature and include olive oil, safflower oil, peanut oil, and corn oil.

Monounsaturated fat. Found in a variety of foods and oils, studies show that eating foods rich in monounsaturated fats improves blood cholesterol levels, which can decrease your risk of disease and produce better health.

Polyunsaturated fat. Found mostly in plant-based foods and oils, eating foods rich in polyunsaturated fats improves blood cholesterol levels, which can decrease risk of heart disease and type 2 diabetes. Omega-3 fatty acids, found in some types of fatty fish, appear to be especially healthy.

That's because some promises are false and because some definitive data are not yet in place, but the goal of this chapter is to provide you with an overview of what we know today.

First, when living with cancer, eating a wholesome diet and maintaining a healthy body weight are priorities. Such lifestyle factors, along with regular physical activity (discussed in the next section), can help maximize the effectiveness of your treatments and help maintain good quality of life, all while minimizing unwanted side effects. In the longer term, they can help reduce your risk of cancer recurrence and your risk of other chronic diseases, and they promote longevity.

As we start our discussion about diet and nutrition, a few guidelines are worth mentioning:

- **No food, vitamin, mineral, or other supplement is going to immediately and miraculously cure your disease or cause you to drop 50 pounds.** That's not to say the benefits of a healthy diet are insignificant, just that eating well is not an immediate fix. To achieve the benefits—and there are many—it takes regular, long-term commitment to a healthier lifestyle. The key is to choose a way of eating that makes the most sense for you, given your personal goals and tastes. Short-term bouts on a healthy diet aren't likely to do much good. But sticking to a healthier diet long term, even if you don't follow it perfectly all the time (moderation is always important!), can make a significant improvement to your health.
- **If you are overweight or obese, weight loss is critical.** The importance of achieving or maintaining a healthy body weight cannot be overstated. Evidence is begin-

ning to accumulate in support of what doctors have long suspected: that losing weight, even after diagnosis, can lead to longer survival. Being overweight is associated with increased risk of recurrence and decreased disease-free survival. Moreover, gaining weight after diagnosis is a frequent complication of treatment, which must be avoided. Managing your weight requires a combination of diet and exercise. It doesn't have to be as daunting as it sounds—the tips in this chapter and the activity chapter will help.

- **Vitamin supplements do not produce the same benefits as diets high in those vitamins.** This has been demonstrated time and again in single-vitamin studies over the past 25 years. Whole-foods diets rich in vegetables, fruits, whole grains, beans, and fish or lean meats, and low in refined sugar, red meat, and high-fat foods, have protective effects against cancer. But the benefits are most likely due to synergistic effects of the many nutrients and phytochemicals present in whole food and not as the result of any one or two nutrients. Supplements can be useful in some cases, such as to meet recommended levels of any vitamins or minerals lacking in your diet, but they cannot replicate the benefits of whole foods. Vitamin D is an example of a nutrient that cancer patients (and others) are frequently deficient in and that may require supplementation (discussed later in this chapter).

- It is **important to make sure you are getting enough protein.** This is important for everyone, but all the more so for cancer patients during all stages of treatment, recovery, and long-term survival. When selecting sources of animal protein, it's best to choose foods that are low in saturated fat, such as fish, lean meat, skinless poultry, eggs, or low-fat dairy. Plant sources of protein, such as beans, nuts, and seeds, have the added benefit of being high in fiber and rich in antioxidants and other healthy plant compounds.

- **Consider seeking individualized nutrition advice.** We all have unique needs, and those of cancer patients are particularly variable depending on the nature of your disease and treatment. As a result, personalized advice can be invaluable. This can be from a doctor who is knowledgeable about nutrition or from a registered dietitian (RD) who has experience with the unique needs of cancer patients. Ask for a referral to an RD who is also a Certified Specialist in Oncology (CSO).

Body Mass Index

Body mass index (BMI) is a good way to determine if you are at a healthy weight or are overweight or obese. There are many free automatic calculators online, such as the U.S. National Institutes of Health website (http://apps.usa.gov/bmi-app.shtml). Simply insert your height and weight in their calculator and your BMI will appear. The website contains information about how to interpret and, if necessary, to reduce your BMI.

Specific Dietary Regimens

In choosing a diet to follow, it's helpful to consider your priorities—whether you need to lose weight or gain it, for instance. Some diets are particularly focused on preventing chronic diseases such as diabetes and heart disease, and that is particularly important if you have a family history of these illnesses or are otherwise at increased risk. And it goes without saying that you'll want to decrease your risk of secondary cancers or recurrences. It's a good idea to consult with a dietitian who can help you consider your options and develop the best plan for you. In this next section, we provide an overview of a few diets that cancer patients may hear about and consider. Some have little, if any, value but are popular among some cancer patients. However, a Mediterranean-type diet is considered by experts as the absolute best so we'll start with that one.

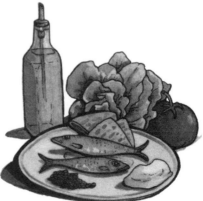

Mediterranean Diet

The Mediterranean diet has become an established eating regimen for decreasing the risk of cancer and its recurrence, as well as the risk of many other chronic diseases. The hallmark of this dietary regimen is low consumption of meat and dairy products. Participants consume fruits, vegetables, legumes (beans, lentils, and the like), and whole grains, with moderate amounts of nuts, seeds, fish, and oils (primarily olive oil). Herbs and spices are generally used in place of salt, and a moderate amount of red wine is consumed with meals. (It must be noted, however, that despite the documented benefits of red wine, alcohol has been shown to increase the risk of certain cancers, so moderation is important.) A recent issue of the *New England Journal of Medicine* was devoted in large part to articles on the Mediterranean diet for prevention of cardiovascular disease. Moreover, the relationship between adherence to the Mediterranean diet and incidence of cancer was studied in a sample of 25,623 people in Greece. At follow-up almost 8 years later, researchers found that better adherence to the diet was associated with lower overall cancer incidence.[5]

Key Components of the *Plant-Based* Mediterranean Diet

- Fruits and vegetables
- Whole grains—breads, pasta, polenta (from corn), bulgur and couscous (from wheat)
- Legumes—beans and lentils
- Seeds and nuts
- Olive oil and other healthy oils
- Fish and poultry
- Red wine once daily

Avoid, or eat rarely, saturated fat from butter, red meat, and eggs. Also avoid deli, luncheon, and cured meats. Eat refined sugars and sweets rarely.

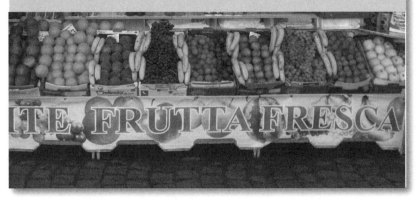

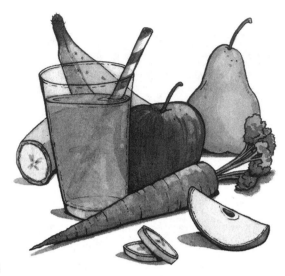

Vegetarian Diets

By definition, a vegetarian diet excludes meat and seafood, emphasizing plant-based foods instead. However, the term "vegetarian" means different things to different people, and as such, vegetarian eating patterns vary widely. Lacto-ovo-vegetarians avoid only meat and seafood, but will eat other animal foods such as dairy and eggs. Lacto-vegetarians exclude eggs in addition to meat and seafood, but consume dairy. Finally, vegans, or total vegetarians, avoid all animal products including dairy and eggs. Other variations exist as well, such as diets that include fish but are otherwise vegan. All vegetarian diets involve significant consumption of whole grains, vegetables, fruit, and beans, including soy products. People often choose plant-based diets out of concern for the environment, for ethical or philosophical reasons (relating to animal welfare), and, increasingly, for their many health benefits.

As long as they are well planned to ensure adequate nutrition, vegetarian diets can be very healthful. The health advantages include lower cholesterol levels and a decreased risk of heart disease, high blood pressure, and type 2 diabetes. Moreover, vegetarians generally have a lower body mass index (BMI) than their meat-eating counterparts and a lower risk of cancer. Vegetarian diets are low in saturated fat and cholesterol (cholesterol is found only in animal foods) and are rich in dietary fiber, minerals such as magnesium and potassium, vitamins C and E, folate, carotenoids (like beta-carotene/vitamin A), flavonoids, and other beneficial phytochemicals. Many of these nutrients are shown to have cancer-protective properties. Consuming them together in the form of whole foods (as compared to individually in dietary supplements) allows them to act in an additive and synergistic manner, maximizing the benefits.

Plant protein can fulfill protein requirements as well as animal protein can, so long as you consume a variety of plant foods each day in sufficient quantities to meet your caloric needs. Together, whole grains and beans consumed in an approximate two-to-one ratio can supply all of the amino acids we need. Calcium requirements, too, can be met through regular consumption of leafy green vegetables, calcium-fortified plant food such as cereals, soy milk, and rice milk, and/or dairy products. Furthermore, diets high in fruit and vegetables help the body hold on to the calcium it already has. The potassium and magnesium content of fruits and vegetables slows loss of calcium from the bones.

However, vegetarian diets can be low in some important nutrients, particularly vitamin B_{12} and vitamin D. It should be noted that humans receive only a very small amount of vitamin D from food. Most vitamin D is obtained from sunlight. However, dark skin and use of sun protector creams, necessary to prevent the deadly skin cancer melanoma, also prevent vitamin D from being synthesized by the body. Therefore, many people are vitamin D deficient. It is worth considering taking a vitamin D supplement to avoid vitamin deficiency. Vitamin B_{12} is found in animal products, including fish, meat, poultry, eggs, milk, and milk products. It is generally not present in plant foods, but fortified breakfast cereals are a readily available source, and supplementation is available.

Vegetarian diets may initially sound dull and boring, but there are many recipes and cookbooks that can help you create attractive, tasty, satisfying, and varied dishes. As more and more people adopt this way of eating, restaurants are increasingly catering to vegetarian and vegan diners as well.

A final note, even those who eat semi-vegetarian diets experience health benefits, so it is not necessary to avoid all animal foods entirely unless you feel inclined to do so.

Dangerous Diets—Some Promoted as Cancer Cures
Macrobiotics
The macrobiotic diet is plant based, comprised largely of whole grains, beans, soups (such as miso soup), and sea veg-

In a 2009 report, the American Dietetic Association concluded that "appropriately planned vegetarian diets, including total vegetarian or vegan diets, are healthful, nutritionally adequate, and may provide health benefits in the prevention and treatment of certain diseases."[6] That said, your nutritional needs may vary compared to the average person, which is why it is important to discuss diet with your doctor and/or another nutrition-trained health professional.

etables. It excludes meat and dairy, but fish is permitted occasionally. Fruits, nuts, and seeds also are consumed at times, along with vegetable pickles and non-caffeinated teas. More than a diet, however, macrobiotics traditionally encompasses both a philosophy and a way of life. It emphasizes balance in the selection, preparation, and consumption of foods, as well as in day-to-day life.

Macrobiotic theory is based largely on the yin-yang principle of balance that was integral to ancient Chinese medicine. Yin and yang are seen to be equal but opposite forces that describe all components of life and the universe. The diet and philosophy were initially developed and popularized by Japanese philosopher George Ohsawa in the early twentieth century. An early disciple, Michio Kushi, led the macrobiotic movement from the mid-1900s. The macrobiotic diet was promoted as a cancer cure in the United States for many years, but that effort eventually waned as scientific studies failed to support the claims.

No diet or combination of foods, in fact, has ever been shown to cure cancer. Moreover, practicing macrobiotics and other extreme diets can lead to nutrient deficiencies, such as vitamin B_{12} and calcium, and inadequate caloric intake.

Gerson Regimen and Metabolic Therapies

Developed in the 1930s by German physician Max Gerson, the Gerson regimen involves a strict metabolic diet, as well as coffee enemas and various supplements intended to aid in detoxifying the body. The diet is vegetarian and emphasizes fresh fruit and vegetable juice; each patient consumes about 20 pounds of fruits and vegetables each day, largely in the form of fresh juice. Supplemental digestive enzymes are frequently given, as well as coffee enemas, which are claimed to stimulate the excretion of bile from the liver and eliminate toxins from the body. This and many other extreme diets are based on the incorrect idea that cancer is caused by a buildup of toxins in the body, and that detoxification will cure the disease. The Gerson clinic advertises its cancer therapy as "a natural treatment that activates the body's extraordinary ability to heal itself through an organic, vegetarian diet, raw juices, coffee enemas, and natural supplements." Along with many other fanciful "therapies" for cancer, the Gerson clinic is located in Tijuana, Mexico, a hotbed of nonviable "alternative" disproved cancer treatments that do not work.

Fasting and Juice Therapies

Fasting eliminates all solid food and generally limits dietary consumption to certain liquids. Juice cleanses or juice fasts, during which only freshly juiced fruits and vegetables are consumed for a period of time that can vary from a few days to weeks, are very common today. Such therapies are promoted for general health maintenance, as well as for healing diseases. Advocates believe they facilitate internal cleansing and support the immune system.

Fresh fruit juice, in moderation, can be healthy as well as delicious. But regimens such as this, especially when continued over an extended period, can be dangerous, especially for cancer patients.

> In summary, eat healthfully; seek professional advice if you have special swallowing or digestive issues; beware of bogus dietary or other cancer "cures"; enjoy the beneficial and delicious Mediterranean-type diet rich in fruits, vegetables, seafood, olive oil, beans, and whole grains.

Important Vitamins and Foods

When researching nutrition for cancer patients online, some vitamin and food entries can create more questions than answers. It is worth spending a bit of time discussing some of those common items.

Soy

Soy can be a confusing
topic for cancer patients.
On the one hand, it is widely
touted as a health food. It contains
compounds called isoflavones,
which may help decrease the
risk of heart disease and
cancer and reduce menopausal symptoms in women, among
other benefits. Soy foods are also an excellent source of plant-
based protein, particularly valuable for vegetarians. As a
result, soy protein is being added to all kinds of processed
foods and is becoming ubiquitous in the food supply.

But the very same isoflavones credited with many of these
benefits are similar in structure to the hormone estrogen.
Doctors and scientists are therefore concerned that they may
mimic estrogen's activity in the human body, potentially encouraging hormone-sensitive tumors (such as estrogen receptor (ER)–positive breast cancer) to grow. So, the question is,
how do these benefits and risks balance out? Is soy something
you should be eating at all, and if so how much is too much?

Soy's journey to mainstream began decades ago, when researchers observed that rates of breast and other cancers were
significantly lower in Asia than in Westernized countries. They
assumed that diet was a factor and zoomed in on soy as a
possible source of this health disparity. Since soy foods were
eaten all the time in Asia but were almost entirely absent from

the Western diet, it seemed a solid hypothesis. Fast-forward 20 years, however, and the research results have been mixed.

Regular consumption of soy foods has been associated with a reduced risk of cancer in many studies, but some laboratory and animal research suggests that soy can promote growth of estrogen-sensitive tumors. It's worth underscoring that virtually all of the studies showing harm were conducted using isolated cells growing in a petrie dish or in rodents—not in humans. And most of them used isolated soy isoflavones, not the soy in its whole-food form. So the degree to which such findings apply to us is not clear. No conclusions can be drawn without considering results in humans.

In recent years, there have been several large public health studies of soy consumption in humans, and all have found it to be safe and perhaps beneficial, even in women with ER-positive breast cancer. Three large studies, two in U.S. breast cancer patients and one in Chinese patients, found no adverse effects of soy consumption on outcome, and suggested it may even offer some protection against recurrence and cancer-related death. The largest of these followed 9,514 U.S. and Chinese breast cancer survivors and found that patients who consumed at least 10 milligrams of isoflavones (about 3 grams of soy protein) per day had a significantly lower risk of cancer recurrence.[7]

Interestingly, it appears that soy is most beneficial when it is eaten regularly early in life and through puberty. Studies suggest that this may decrease the risk of breast cancer, but that introducing soy into the diets of adult women may not do much to change their cancer risk, either positively or negatively.

The bottom line, considering all of the findings so far, is that eating moderate amounts of soy should be fine. In its most recent set of guidelines, the American Cancer Society concluded that for breast cancer patients "current evidence suggests no adverse effects on recurrence or survival from consuming soy and soy foods."

That said, it is wise to avoid supplements that contain high doses of isolated soy isoflavones. Stick to soy-containing foods, such as miso soup, tofu, tempeh, soymilk, edamame, and even soybeans in their original form.

Vitamin D

Vitamin D is a fat-soluble vitamin (technically a hormone precursor) that is produced in our skin when exposed to sunlight, and is 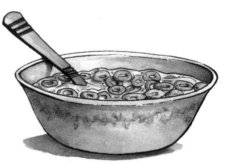 also found in plants, fish, and dairy products. Its effects in the body are widespread: thousands of genes are regulated directly or indirectly by vitamin D. Scientists know that it is important for bone formation and that it assists in the absorption of calcium; adequate vitamin D levels are necessary to prevent osteoporosis and bone fractures. Although far more equivocal, some studies suggest that vitamin D may play a role in cancer, cardiovascular disease, diabetes, physical functioning, autoimmune diseases, infections/immune function, and mental health, among other diseases. Many argue that vitamin D supplementation can prevent or improve these conditions. But study results have been mixed, and evidence is lacking for virtually all uses except bone health.

Our need for this vitamin is not surprising; through most of human evolution, vitamin D was readily available. Our hunter-gatherer ancestors spent most of their time outside in the sun and presumably produced high levels of vitamin D. But our modern indoors lifestyle has made vitamin D deficiency a widespread problem. Deficiency is even more prevalent among darker-skinned people, who make less vitamin D to begin with than their lighter-skinned counterparts.

Of particular relevance for this book, there is limited but promising evidence that vitamin D may have a role in decreasing the risk or progression of some cancers. While vitamin D supplementation has not been shown to improve outcomes in cancer patients, some studies, especially those involving colon cancer, are suggestive of anticancer effects.[8] However, the numerous efforts to delineate a causal relationship between vitamin D and a wide array of human cancers have produced conflicting results, and large-scale randomized trials will be required to provide definitive answers.[9]

Large portions of the population, including many cancer patients, are deficient in vitamin D. Even though improvements in outcome from taking vitamin D after diagnosis have yet to be documented, correcting a deficiency is generally considered to be safe and worthwhile. The best way to increase your intake of vitamin D is through oral supplements, which are widely available. Although spending more time in the sun will increase your vitamin D levels, it also increases your risk of skin cancer. Wearing sunscreen, which blocks ultraviolet (UV) rays from being absorbed by your skin, also blocks vitamin D synthesis.

Ideally, have a doctor check your levels with a simple blood test so they can help you choose the right supplemental dosage, if needed. The current Dietary Allowance recommended by the Institute of Medicine is 600 IU per day (800 IU per day for persons over 70 years), but many people require much more than that in order to maintain an adequate blood level of the vitamin. A blood level of 20 ng/mL or less is classified as a deficiency; a sufficient level is generally agreed to be 30 ng/mL or higher. Some experts advise that 1,500 to 2,000 IU per day of vitamin D (for adults) is needed to achieve the optimal blood level. However, the amount needed varies greatly for different people.

Antioxidants

Antioxidants help to prevent cellular damage by neutralizing free radicals, unstable molecules that are produced through your body's normal metabolic activity. Exposure

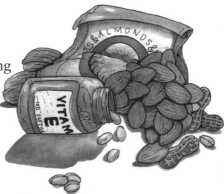

to radiation and tobacco smoke, among other environmental factors, may also generate free radicals. Once formed, they can damage your DNA, creating mutations that may lead to cancer. On this basis, scientists have theorized that a diet rich in antioxidants may help to prevent cancer.

Many observational studies in humans in fact suggest that people who eat more vegetables and fruits high in antioxidants, such as vitamin C, vitamin E, and beta-carotene, have a lower chance of getting certain cancers. Of course, antioxidant content is just one of many reasons that it is wise to eat a variety of vegetables and fruit every day. Antioxidants in pill form produce mixed results and are not as effective as dietary intake.

Three major studies of beta-carotene supplementation, involving a total of 74,000 people, found no effect on cancer risk. Alarmingly, however, a study of 540 head and neck cancer patients undergoing radiation treatment found a higher rate of death among those taking 400 IU of vitamin E each day compared to placebo.[10]

That said, there is not strong enough evidence to draw solid conclusions about the risks and benefits of most antioxidant supplements. Most of the existing studies are of relatively low quality or limited statistical power. Variations in the types of cancer studied, as well as the types and doses of antioxidants used, further complicate matters and make it difficult to compare studies.

It's also not entirely clear how antioxidant supplements could cause harm. One theory has to do with dose: at high doses, some antioxidants can become pro-oxidants, meaning they promote free radical damage. Another possibility is that some amount of free radicals is needed for the body's immune system to function properly, and that mopping those all up with high-dose antioxidants could cause problems. Or, there could be some other explanation for these results. Until more is known, the safest bet is to focus on eating a wholesome diet, with plenty of colorful vegetables and fruit. The latest guidelines from the American Cancer Society point out that this is particularly important for cancer patients as it may help to reduce the risk of secondary cancers.

It is wise not to consume antioxidant supplements during chemotherapy or radiation, however, unless your doctor advises you otherwise. Since some of these therapies attack cancer cells by producing free radicals, antioxidants can potentially interfere by protecting cancer cells as well as normal ones from damage. At other times, such as before and after treatment, some antioxidant supplements at reasonable doses may have value. Consult with a healthcare professional first and be sure you are not taking an excessive amount.

Vitamin C

Vitamin C (ascorbic acid) is a particularly popular antioxidant. It is a water-soluble vitamin found in citrus fruits, such as oranges, as well as in other fresh fruits and vegetables. It is commonly taken as a dietary supplement for immune stimulation, wound healing, and for prevention of heart disease and cancer. Although the vitamin has been found to reduce the severity and duration of respiratory infections, evidence is lacking for its use in prevention of chronic diseases such as cancer.

Based on the work of Nobel laureate Linus Pauling in the 1970s, megadoses of vitamin C have been claimed to extend the lives of or possibly cure patients with advanced cancer, but there is no evidence supporting its use for this purpose. In several clinical trials, orally administered high-dose vitamin C failed to extend survival or otherwise benefit end-stage cancer patients. Three of these studies, conducted by Mayo Clinic researchers, orally administered 10 grams of vitamin C per day to patients with advanced cancer and found no benefit over the placebo group, which received sugar pills in place of vitamin C.[11]

More recently, however, some studies have suggested that high-dose vitamin C may be more effective when administered intravenously, presumably because this leads to higher blood concentrations of the vitamin. Several clinical trials are in the works to assess the safety and efficacy of this approach for treating cancer. Meanwhile, however, high-dose vitamin C must be considered an unproven approach to cancer treatment, with potentially serious negative risks. Note that supplemental vitamin C, as with other antioxidant vitamins, may decrease the effectiveness of many chemotherapy drugs and should be avoided during the course of treatment unless your oncologist advises otherwise.

Sugar

According to U.S. Department of Agriculture estimates, the average American eats somewhere between 80 and 130 pounds of sugar each year. It comes in many forms, from regular table sugar to high-fructose corn syrup to "natural" sweeteners such as molasses or honey. Although we commonly associate sugar with sodas, candy, and junk food, it's also added to just about every processed food you can imagine, from bread and pasta sauce to peanut butter. Health-food store brands are no exception. Although such items may use sugar in its natural form, like cane juice or raw sugar, rather than high-fructose corn syrup (HFCS), the effects on our bodies are much the same.

Sugar consumption has not yet been shown to directly increase the risk or progression of cancer, but there are plenty of reasons to avoid sweet foods as much as possible. A high-sugar diet contributes to weight gain, which in turn is associated with poorer cancer outcomes. Sweet foods provide a lot of calories, but not much nutrition. Worse, they often take the place of more nutritious foods in our diets: eating a candy bar after work may make you less likely to finish that bowl of vegetables at dinner. Diets rich in sugar can also increase your risk of other chronic diseases, such as diabetes and heart disease.

Intriguing research points to a particular type of sugar, fructose, as uniquely problematic. Fructose is metabolized in a different way than its fellow sugars, and excessive consumption of it appears to bring on a condition known as metabolic syndrome. This syndrome is increasingly common around the world, and usually presents as a combination of obesity, insulin resistance, and inflammation. It puts you on the road to diabetes and heart disease. Moreover, metabolic syndrome has been shown to worsen the prognosis of breast cancer (the same likely applies to other cancers as well). So what is fructose, where is it found, and why might it be so bad?

First, a quick primer on different types of sugar and where fructose fits in. All sugars are comprised of molecules called monosaccarides, which are simple sugars that essentially act as the building blocks of more complex sugars. The simple sugars include glucose, galactose, and fructose. Glucose is the most basic source of energy for all of the cells in your body; anything you eat can be converted into glucose to feed your cells. Glucose and galactose together form lactose, which is the sugar found in milk. And fructose is the simple sugar that's naturally found in fruit. It's also found in table sugar (sucrose) and high-fructose corn syrup (HFCS). Both of these are made up of about half fructose and half glucose. The main difference between table sugar and HFCS is where it comes from: sucrose is typically extracted from sugar cane or beets, whereas HFCS is made from corn through an enzymatic process. HFCS is worse in the sense that it is found in high quantity in more foods (because it's cheaper than sucrose), but its fructose content and effect on the body are more or less the same.

The issue with fructose, and by extension table sugar and high-fructose corn syrup, is the way our bodies metabolize it. Unlike glucose, which can be directly absorbed and utilized by all of our cells, fructose must first be changed into glucose by the liver. When the liver is overloaded with fructose, it begins to change it into liver fat instead. Excess liver fat appears to underlie weight gain, metabolic syndrome, and the downstream chronic health effects.

The bottom line here is that not all calories (or carbs) are created equal. We've long thought that eating 1,500 calories in a day and burning 2,000 through daily activities and exercise, for example, would lead to weight loss. But newer science shows that losing weight and getting healthier may not be as simple as eating fewer calories than you expend each day. It's not just how much you eat, but what you eat. Foods that are low in sugar, particularly added sugar, and high in fiber and other nutrients are the way to go. This is essentially the secret behind successful diets. A serving of beans, let's say, that is high in fiber, packed with nutrients, and low in sugar, is far better for you than a calorically equivalent amount of soda or even orange juice. To whatever extent possible, you should choose real, whole foods over processed foods. If it has more than one ingredient, it's a processed food.

A Note about Supplements

Dietary supplements are widely used. Over half of U.S. adults and close to 81 percent of cancer survivors take dietary supplements. Up to a third of cancer survivors start using supplements after their diagnosis. A nutritionally healthy diet is essential to overall good health, and sometimes vitamin and mineral supplements are required to meet nutritional needs. But research over the past 25 years strongly suggests that dietary supplements cannot replace the value of a wholesome and nutritionally complete diet. The research results are mixed, but in most studies taking isolated vitamins and minerals had little or no effect on disease outcome, and in a few cases even led to harm.

The use of vitamins, minerals, and other supplements during the course of cancer treatment is particularly controversial, and most oncologists advise against it. Doctors are particularly concerned about supplements that act as antioxidants (such as beta-carotene, vitamin A, vitamin C, and selenium, among others). These help to repair cellular damage caused by free radicals. But the relatively high doses found in many supplements could potentially decrease the effectiveness of chemotherapy or radiation therapy by protecting cancer cells as well as healthy cells from damage.

However, other experts argue the opposite—that antioxidant supplementation could selectively protect healthy cells from such damage, thus minimizing toxicity of the treatment. Until further study clears up the issue, it is wise to be cautious. The American Cancer Society advises that cancer patients try to consume antioxidants and other nutrients through food rather than dietary supplements whenever possible. Whole food contains a broad mix of nutrients and other plant chemicals that may act synergistically to promote health, without any risks that may come from isolated nutrients in pill form.

Supplements may be safer and potentially more helpful after your treatment is completed. It is critical, however, that you tell your doctor what supplements you are taking at any given point, to ensure that you are not taking something that could reduce the effectiveness of your treatment.

A Note about Herbs

Herbs and other botanicals have been used as medicines since the beginning of human history. They contain biologically active compounds that can have a significant effect on bodily functions—for better or for worse. About 40 percent of the prescription medications available today—including some major cancer drugs—were originally derived from herbs found in nature. For example, vincristine and vinblastine, used to treat hematologic (blood) cancers, were derived from a species of rosy periwinkle found in Madagascar. Irinotecan and topotecan, also used to combat cancer, were partly derived from the Chinese Happy Tree (*Camptotheca acuminate*). Taxol and other taxanes, used to treat breast cancer and other malignancies, are derived from the bark of the Pacific yew tree.

That said, it is critical to understand that "natural" does not always mean "safe." Plants can be health promoting, but they can also be poisonous. Eating a single castor bean, for example, can be fatal. Similarly, it is tempting to think that herbs and other natural products are safe and effective simply because they have been used over the millennia. When studied with the tools of modern science, many turn out to be ineffective or even harmful. Herbs are unrefined pharmaceuticals, and we must understand their power and remain cautious in their use.

Just as people on prescription medications are concerned about drug-drug interactions, oncologists and their patients must also be concerned with herb-drug interactions. Garlic, ginseng, ginkgo, and vitamin E can interfere with blood coagulation. American ginseng lowers blood sugar, and Saint-John's-wort, valerian, and many other herbs decrease the activity of prescription medications including chemotherapy drugs. Kava can cause liver failure, and many herbs can bring about gastrointestinal problems, liver toxicity, or kidney toxicity.

Memorial Sloan-Kettering Cancer Center (MSKCC) has developed a website and free app containing everything you need to know about herbs and other dietary supplements. Visit MSKCC.org/AboutHerbs for more information or to download the free app.

Herbal supplements may also be beneficial in certain circumstances. Despite some conflicting data, echinacea may reduce the duration of the common cold, black cohosh may help treat menopausal symptoms, and the chief active ingredient in green tea, called EGCG, may help to reduce the risk of cancer or cancer recurrence. Like other dietary supplements, however, most oncologists warn against the use of herbal supplements at least during chemotherapy or radiation treatment. Some herbs, similarly to certain vitamins and minerals, have antioxidant activity and may interfere with the effectiveness of cancer treatments. Many herbs also have components that act similar to estrogen in the human body and can potentially promote growth of hormone-sensitive malignancies, such as ER-positive breast cancer.

Again, the best way to make sure you're not putting yourself at risk is to discuss any herbal supplements you are taking, or are thinking about taking, with a physician or other cancer care professional knowledgeable in herb-drug interactions.

Where Do I Get Started?

Healthy food options can be found in any supermarket that offers high-quality produce, whole grains, etc. Supplements and herbal remedies are available in pill and liquid form in health food stores, at some pharmacies, and all over the Internet. No diet has been shown to cure cancer—though a healthy one that emphasizes fruits, vegetables, whole grains, and lean animal foods can promote general wellness, reduce the risk of cancer, maintain strength during cancer treatment, and help prevent recurrence.

In this section we have provided many general guidelines, but your nutritional needs may vary depending on your specific disease and course of treatment. For personalized advice, ask your doctor to refer you to a registered dietitian who is also a certified specialist in oncology (CSO), meaning they are trained to work with cancer patients and experienced in developing nutritional plans to meet your unique needs.

Notes

1. Richman EL, Kenfield SA, Chavarro JE, et al. Fat intake after diagnosis and risk of lethal prostate cancer and all-cause mortality. *JAMA Intern Med.* 2013 Jul 22;173(14):1318–26.

2. Makarem N, Chandran U, Bandera EV, Parekh N. Dietary fat in breast cancer survival. *Annu Rev Nutr.* 2013 Jul 17;33:319–48.

3. Wolin KY, Colditz GA. Cancer and beyond: healthy lifestyle choices for cancer survivors. *J Natl Cancer Inst.* 2013 May 1;105(9):593–4.

4. www.mayoclinic.com/health/fat/nu00262/nsectiongroup=2

5. V Benetou, A Trichopoulou, P Orfanos, et al. Conformity to traditional Mediterranean diet and cancer incidence: the Greek EPIC cohort. *Br J Cancer.* 2008;99:191–195.

6. http://www.ncbi.nlm.nih.gov/pubmed/19562864

7. Kang X, Zhang Q, Wang S, Huang X, Jin S. Effect of soy isoflavones on breast cancer recurrence and death for patients receiving adjuvant endocrine therapy. *CMAJ.* 2010 Nov 23;182(17):1857–62.

8. Ma Y, Zhang P, Wang F, Yang J, Liu Z, Qin H. Association between vitamin D and risk of colorectal cancer: a systematic review of prospective studies. *J Clin Oncol.* 2011 Oct 1;29(28):3775–82.

9. Kennel KA, Drake MT. Vitamin D in the cancer patient. *Curr Opin Support Palliat Care.* 2013 Sep;7(3):272–7.

10. Bairati I, Meyer F, Jobin E, et al. Antioxidant vitamins supplementation and mortality: a randomized trial in head and neck cancer patients. *Int J Cancer.* 2006 Nov 1;119(9):2221–4.

11. Moertel CG, Fleming TR, Creagan ET, Rubin J, O'Connell MJ, Ames MM. High-dose vitamin C versus placebo in the treatment of patients with advanced cancer who have had no prior chemotherapy. A randomized double-blind comparison. *N Engl J Med.* 1985 Jan 17;312(3):137–41.

Worksheet 1: My Medications and Supplements

The following table can help you to keep track of any prescription medicines, over-the-counter medicines, and herbs, vitamins, or other dietary supplements you are taking. You can bring this to the doctor's office with you.

Medication	Times Taken	Dose / Prescribed by	Recommended/ Reason	Side Effects

Visit www.sprypubcancer.com to download a printable sheet.

Physical Activity

Our bodies were made to move, yet modern life has become very sedentary. We spend our working hours at desks and our leisure hours on couches, often staring at computer screens or TVs. We get from place to place by riding in cars, or buses, or trains. And the amount of time we devote to walking, running, or any other physical activity is a mere fraction of what it once was.

Incorporating activity into your life, however, is not as daunting as it may sound. The benefits, particularly for cancer patients, are simply too great to overlook. Physical activity enhances our bodies and sharpens our minds. It reduces our risk of serious chronic problems, such as heart disease, diabetes, and cancer, while combating fatigue, anxiety, and depression. Moreover, it may extend our lives: a recent National Institutes of Health study found that people who were most physically active in their free time lived up to four and a half years longer than those who were least active. Any amount of exercise, no matter how small, was associated with improvements in lifespan.[1]

Benefits of Exercise

Exercise can make you thinner, stronger, and fitter, while also helping you fight depression, fatigue, and disease. It also increases life span.

Physical Benefits
- Increased cardiovascular fitness
- Greater muscle strength
- Reduced risk of cardiovascular disease and diabetes

Psychological Benefits
- Improved mood
- More self-confidence and self-esteem
- Increased happiness
- Reduced fatigue

For patients already diagnosed with cancer, exercise is just as important, if not more so. A flood of recent studies shows that cancer patients who are more physically active tend to live longer after their diagnosis and are at decreased risk of the cancer coming back. The numbers are truly remarkable. One observational study of 933 women with breast cancer found that 2.5 hours per week of brisk walking or other moderate-intensity exercise—the level recommended for the general population by the U.S. Department of Health and Human services—was associated with a 67 percent lower risk of death compared to inactive women. A recent analysis that pooled the results of six other studies found that those who exercised after diagnosis had a lower risk of death from cancer, a lower risk of death from any cause, and a lower risk of breast cancer recurrence.[2]

So far these findings are limited to breast, colorectal,

prostate, and ovarian cancer, but there is good reason to believe that the benefits of exercise will hold true for other cancers as well. Further study is rapidly ongoing.

Moreover, exercise is safe and practical both during and after treatment. In other words, physical activity—to whatever extent you can manage—can benefit you at any stage of your disease and treatment. Exercise can help your body defend against cancer, allowing you to lead a longer, healthier life. If you haven't already, now is the time to jump on the exercise bandwagon. It is perhaps the single most important self-care strategy for long-term health.

Some important points to consider:

- **Engage in some kind of physical activity every day.** It can be as simple as walking for a half hour each day, or something more intense if you are able and so inclined. If you live near a park or wooded area, walking, jogging, or gardening also provides a healthful opportunity to reconnect with nature. A growing body of research finds that exposure to nature can decrease stress and improve your memory and attention span, among other benefits. The established recommendation of the U.S. Department of Health and Human Services is that adults age 18 to 64 engage in regular aerobic physical activity of moderate intensity for at least 2.5 hours per week or of vigorous intensity for 1.25 hours per week. This should be your goal.
- **Start exercising as soon as possible after diagnosis.**

Stress, depression, and other symptoms of cancer may make it harder to motivate yourself to be active, but it is critical to fight that impulse. Exercising combats these symptoms and will help you to break out of the downward spiral and boost your recovery. If you weren'tvery active before diagnosis, you'll have to start slow—and that's okay. Talk to your doctor or seek out an exercise instructor who has experience with cancer patients to decide on the best way to get started.

- **Exercise will have the greatest long-term impact when combined with a healthy diet.** As we mentioned in the diet section, breast cancer patients who ate five or more daily servings of vegetables and fruit and took part in physical activity equivalent to 30 minutes of walking six days per week had a higher survival rate, more so than for either diet or exercise alone. One step at a time, but don't forget that changing your lifestyle for the better includes both diet and exercise.

The U.S. Department of Health and Human Services recommends that adults get at least 150 minutes of moderate intensity exercise (i.e., brisk walking) per week and muscle strengthening exercises on 2 or more days. For more information, visit www.cdc.gov/physicalactivity/everyone/guidelines.

Exercise is a huge topic, so this chapter tackles only what we feel is most relevant for people fighting cancer. We first review the effects of physical activity in general, and then address specific kinds of exercise. Finally, we conclude with some important tips and precautions.

Cancer Survival and Recurrence

Exercise is unique among complementary therapies in that its proven benefits go beyond symptom control and quality of life improvements. Like acupuncture, meditation, and massage, physical activity is a tool that may help minimize your symptoms and enhance your overall well-being, but in addition, it can actually extend your life. More than 20 large observational studies to date have shown that physically active cancer survivors have a lower risk of recurrence and ultimately live longer than those who are inactive. First the evidence began piling up for breast cancer patients, and then for colorectal cancer patients, and most recently for prostate and ovarian cancer patients. Additional study is needed, but it is very likely that the benefits of exercise will hold true for other cancers as well. Moreover, this research demonstrates that exercise is safe for cancer patients, even during treatment. Along with a healthy diet, exercise is probably the best thing you can do for yourself to promote long-term health, and it can be beneficial even if you've never entered a gym or lifted a weight until after your diagnosis.

The data consistently show exercise to be associated with a reduced risk of cancer recurrence and increased survival. For breast cancer patients who exercise, a decreased mortality risk of 40–67 percent was observed across studies. The more patients exercised (within reason!), the lower their risk of death. Because individual

> All integrative therapies help *add life to your years,* but exercise (along with a healthy diet) may actually *add years to your life.*

studies may have too few participants to draw strong conclusions, scientists sometimes perform a meta-analysis, meaning they combine the raw data from several different studies together in order to test the strength of the results. Such efforts have further confirmed the survival advantage of those who exercise. A recent meta-analysis that pooled the results of six other studies, covering 12,108 breast cancer patients in all, found that those who exercised after diagnosis had a 34 percent lower risk of death from cancer, a 41 percent lower risk of death from any cause, and a 24 percent lower risk of breast cancer recurrence.[3]

With colon cancer patients, the findings are equally promising. Several large studies in colorectal cancer survivors have documented improvements of up to 50 percent in survival and recurrence risk in patients who engaged in physical activity after diagnosis. Based on the promise of these findings, a gold-standard randomized controlled trial called the Colon Health and Life-Long Exercise Change trial (CHALLENGE) is now underway to assess the effects of a 3-year physical activity program on clinical outcomes in Stage II and III colon cancer survivors who have completed chemotherapy.

Similarly promising evidence is beginning to build up in

support of post-diagnosis exercise for prostate and ovarian cancer patients, and as more studies are conducted, it is very likely to hold true for other cancer diagnoses as well.

The bottom line is that exercise can bring great benefit to cancer patients with little risk of harm. Research is ongoing and will eventually facilitate more specific exercise guidelines for cancer patients, such as the most effective amount, timing, and type of exercise. In the meantime, the best advice for cancer patients is to meet the U.S. government's recommendation of 2.5 hours per week of moderate exercise, to the extent your physical condition allows. There are important precautions, however. To minimize the risk of exercise-related injuries or other adverse effects, it's important that you choose an exercise plan that takes into account your physical condition and treatment regimen, among other factors. For example, you must be particularly cautious if you have weak bones or are at risk for or have osteoporosis. Talk to your doctor, who can help you choose an appropriate exercise plan or direct you to an exercise professional with experience in this area.

How Does Activity Promote Survival?

Although the specific mechanisms that bridge the gap between exercise and cancer outcomes are not yet well understood, we do know that exercise can have many broad effects on our bodies. These effects go far beyond increasing our physical strength and range from increasing our mental capacity to helping us fight diseases such as heart disease and cancer.

Broadly, physical activity can regulate metabolism and positively affect our biochemistry. It can decrease body fat, modulate levels of hormones such as insulin and estrogen, reduce inflammation, boost the immune system, and promote a process of cellular cleanup called autophagy.

Each of these physiologic results and how physical activity regulates metabolism and improves our biochemistry and our health are discussed in more detail in the following sections.

Body Fat and Insulin Levels

Exercise, particularly when combined with a healthy diet, can help you to lose weight and combat a group of health conditions known as metabolic syndrome. This condition is a combination of medical disorders that frequently occur together, including overweight/obesity (particularly extra weight around the middle and upper body), insulin resistance, and inflammation. It puts you at increased risk of heart attack, stroke, and type 2 diabetes and may worsen cancer prognosis. Unfortunately, metabolic syndrome is becoming increasingly common in the United States, probably driven by lifestyle factors such as poor diet and inadequate exercise. While it often involves weight problems, even people who are not overweight can have metabolic syndrome and face the associated risks.

Research in breast cancer patients shows that those who suffer from metabolic syndrome have worse outcomes. A study of 512 non-diabetic breast cancer patients found that those with the highest fasting insulin levels at time of diagnosis fared the worst, with double the risk of disease recurrence and death.[4]

Here's a more detailed look at three of the more problematic metabolic issues:

- **Insulin resistance.** Insulin is a hormone that helps regulate blood sugar. When you eat a meal, your pancreas secretes insulin into the blood, which in turn signals cells all over your body to take up glucose from the bloodstream. This normal process gets your cells the energy they need while keeping your blood sugar in check.

  Over time, however, eating a sugary diet requires so much insulin that your cells start to become insulin resistant. They don't respond as efficiently to insulin, so it takes even more of it to get the job done. Accordingly, your pancreas has to work harder and your body experiences significant spikes and swings in blood sugar, particularly after meals. This inability to properly regulate blood sugar is detrimental and brings on type 2 diabetes. It has also been linked to cardiovascular disease and is one component of the broader metabolic syndrome that may promote poorer cancer outcomes.

  Clinical studies show, however, that regular physical activity promotes insulin sensitivity and leads to beneficial changes in the level of circulating insulin and insulin-like growth factor 1 (IGF-1). Exercise essentially helps your cells to more efficiently utilize energy from your food while keeping blood sugar down. This is just one of many benefits of physical activity that goes beyond the number of calories you burn.

- **Inflammation.** Inflammation is a critical part of the body's healing response. It can appear as redness, heat, and swelling at the site of an injury or infection. It brings increased blood flow and therefore more white blood cells and other immune factors to the affected area.

Despite these benefits, however, the inflammatory response can sometimes go awry. Chronic inflammation in your body may be one factor that promotes cancer progression and other diseases. Research suggests that inflammation surrounding a tumor may help to drive angiogenesis, the process by which cancers recruit blood supplies, and metastasis, the process by which tumors spread. A recent study in mice with human breast tumors demonstrated that increased inflammatory signaling in tissue surrounding the tumor led to faster cancer growth. Moreover, disruption of this signaling caused impaired growth.

Exercise may help regulate and minimize this sort of chronic inflammation. Researchers have studied inflammation in humans who exercise by measuring their blood levels of C-reactive protein (CRP). CRP is a marker of general inflammation in the body; the more CRP in your blood, the more inflammation

(though it doesn't indicate where specifically the inflammation is occurring). Exercise in some breast cancer and prostate cancer studies was shown to decrease
circulating CRP levels. Whether this particular factor
has a meaningful effect on risk of cancer recurrence
or survival remains unknown, but this is possible and
maybe even likely. Further research will help to parse
out cause and effect.

- **Weight loss.** Studies show that being overweight or
obese increases the likelihood of cancer recurrence and
decreases chances for disease-free survival. Perhaps
more importantly, studies are beginning to confirm
that, for those who are overweight, intentionally losing
weight after diagnosis may lead to better outcomes.
Maintaining a healthy weight and avoiding weight gain
after a cancer diagnosis are of critical importance, not
only for their ability to improve long-term prognosis,
but also to improve quality of life and physical fitness.

Thus, weight loss facilitated by exercise may help
cancer patients live longer. Although exercise will
make you healthier, it's important to remember that
it alone may not lead to significant changes in your
overall weight. Weight loss usually requires both
dietary and exercise changes.

While the conventional wisdom is that we lose
weight when we eat less and exercise more, that may
not be the whole story, as discussed in the diet chapter.

Put simply, a calorie is not a calorie. Calories from certain foods may lead to more weight gain and are less healthy than calories from other foods. That is, some foods can have a greater fattening potential per calorie than others. Avoiding specific kinds of foods, such as sugar and refined grains, can be particularly helpful.

A long-term study of 120,877 healthy men and women conducted by scientists at Harvard, for example, analyzed the impact of many lifestyle factors on weight and supports this point. Foods that lead to the most weight gain include French fries, potato chips, and other forms of potatoes, sugar-sweetened drinks, red meats and processed meats, sweets and desserts, refined grains, fried foods, fruit juice, and butter.

Those who slept for fewer than six hours, or more than eight hours a night, generally gained weight as well. Not surprisingly, those who consumed more fruits, vegetables, and whole grains (and less refined grains, sugar, and meat) tended to lose, or at least not to gain, weight. The same was true for exercise.[5]

All of this said, actively pursuing weight loss during your initial course of treatment can be challenging and stressful. It is not unreasonable to put this off until after the initial treatment phase. But it is very important that you try to avoid gaining weight, a problem that plagues many cancer patients. If you do want to focus on losing weight during treatment, make sure to discuss this with your doctor. In general, moderate weight loss is helpful and likely to have significant health benefits, even if you don't fully achieve your ideal weight. It's also worth noting that the advice in this section does not apply to patients with certain types of cancer that may lead to extreme weight loss, such as some head and neck or digestive system tumors. In these cases, maitaining a healthy weight may require increased intake of nutrients and calories. In general, be sure to discuss any exercise and dietary plans with your healthcare provider.

Sex Hormone Levels

The hormone estrogen plays an important role in the development and progression of estrogen receptor (ER)–positive breast cancer. For example, studies show that a relatively high level of circulating estrogen in postmenopausal women greatly increases breast cancer risk. Moreover, decreasing the production and/or activity of estrogen in the body lowers the risk of breast cancer and breast cancer recurrences in women already diagnosed. In fact, a common breast cancer drug, tamoxifen, works by blocking estrogen receptors, essentially minimizing the hormone's effects. Another class of drugs called aromatase inhibitors brings about a similar effect by blocking the body's natural production of estrogen.

Research suggests that exercise may also help to reduce estrogen levels. Some studies show that women with ER-positive tumors who exercised had better survival rates than women with other forms of breast cancer who exercised about the same amount. Since the ER-positive tumors are fueled by estrogen, exercise may work in part by decreasing the amount of active estrogen in the body. Further research will be needed to confirm—and explain—this phenomenon. Because fat tissue releases estrogen and is the primary source of sex hormones after menopause, it is possible that exercise decreases estrogen levels simply by promoting weight loss. With less fat, there would presumably be less estrogen production. Regardless, the bottom line is that the benefits of physical activity, at least for breast cancer patients, may include positive hormonal effects.

Immune System

Cancer is associated with negative changes to immune function. In healthy people, the immune system helps protect against cancer by recognizing and destroying abnormal cells that might otherwise produce a tumor. As such, it is possible that improvements in immune function could favorably affect prognosis and improve survival. Some research in breast cancer survivors suggests that moderate physical activity may do just that. A few small studies show that exercise can boost the immune system, increasing the activity of various kinds of white blood cells. This includes natural killer (NK) cells, which the body uses to destroy abnormal or cancerous cells. Although additional and larger studies are needed to confirm these effects, increased immune system activity provides another plausible explanation for the benefits of physical activity in cancer survivors.

Autophagy

Recent research suggests that exercise may promote a cellular recycling program called autophagy. Derived from the Greek for "self-eating," autophagy is a process in which damaged cell components, such as organelles and proteins, are collected and degraded so their building blocks can be reused. Much as our homes collect clutter over time, our cells accumulate a variety of debris from everyday processes, including damaged proteins, pieces of cell membrane, harmful microbes, and other worn-out cellular machinery. Through autophagy, all of this garbage is rounded up, wrapped in a membrane, and carried to a cellular compartment called the lysosome where it is broken down. The resulting pieces are used either to build new cellular structures or as a food source for energy.

This process of cellular renewal is critical; without this ability to eliminate waste and reuse worn parts, cells cannot function as efficiently or, eventually, at all. Scientists suspect that diminished autophagy as we get older may contribute to aging, and that faulty autophagy may play some role in the development of health problems from diabetes to Alzheimer's disease and even cancer.

A 2012 study published in the leading journal *Nature* convincingly showed that exercise induces autophagy in mice. Scientists at the University of Texas (UT) Southwestern Medical Center used two groups of running mice. The first batch of animals had been genetically engineered so that the membranes involved in autophagy would glow green. After half an hour of running, the mice had significantly more of these membranes in their muscles, indicating an increased rate of autophagy. Previous laboratory studies had found that autophagy speeds up when cells are starved or otherwise stressed, and exercise is a form of physiological stress.

To find out whether increased autophagy had any biological significance, the UT Southwestern Medical Center researchers then created a second group of mice with genetic alterations that prevent them from responding to exercise in this way. Although these new mice had normal levels of autophagy at baseline, exercise could not increase the rate. When this second, autophagy-resistant group of mice ran alongside their normal counterparts, they became fatigued much more quickly and their muscles were less efficient at gathering sugar from the bloodstream.

Moreover, when the researchers fed both groups of mice a diet designed to cause diabetes, the normal mice were able to reverse the disease by running whereas the autophagy-resistant mice remained diabetic even after weeks of exercise. They also had higher cholesterol than the normal mice.[6]

Thus, autophagy appears to be a critical means through which exercise improves health. Put another way, the benefits of exercise depend, at least in part, on its ability to boost the rate of autophagy. It remains to be determined whether or to what degree increased autophagy can specifically explain the life-extending effects of exercise—but this exciting new area of research points strongly to a likely mechanism behind at least some of the protective benefits of regular exercise.

Types of Exercise and Their Benefits

As we discussed, the more physically active you are, the greater the beneficial effects. But even a little activity, practiced regularly, can go a long way, and our bodies actually respond to exercise very quickly. Consider a recent study conducted at the University of Missouri, for example. To look at the impact of inactivity on health, researchers assigned healthy, active volunteers to significantly decrease their levels of exercise. Subjects had to reduce the number of steps they took daily by half, for a period of 3 days. In that short period of time, the volunteers' blood sugar levels began to spike significantly after meals, with the peaks growing higher each successive day. If inactivity were to continue over the long term, such a state could bring on obesity, diabetes, and other chronic diseases. But add regular physical activity back in, and things revert to their healthier state. Exercise alone, of course, is not enough to guarantee good health—diet and other factors are clearly important as well. But being sedentary may be one of the worst things we can do to ourselves.[7]

Jim, age 58 with lung cancer, following weeks of exercise class attendance

"I wanted to get off the inhaler. I am completely off of it after working with [the exercise therapist] and today I climbed 5 flights of stairs."

That said, there's no need to join a gym or become a work-out fanatic. Becoming active can be as simple as brisk walking for 20 to 30 minutes per day, or you can incorporate any combination of other activities. You can bike, dance, swim, or do anything else that gets you up and moving. Choose things that are fun for you or that you enjoy doing with other people. Exercising with others tends to be more rewarding than doing

Moderate and Vigorous Activities

The U.S. Department of Health and Human Services recommends that you engage in moderate-intensity exercise for 150 minutes or vigorous intensity-exercise for 75 minutes each week (or an equivalent combination of the two), but what does that mean? The chart that follows gives examples of activities that meet the criteria for both "moderate" and "vigorous" exercise.

Moderate Activities
(I can talk while I do them, but I can't sing.)

- Ballroom and line dancing
- Biking on level ground or with few hills
- Canoeing
- General gardening (raking, trimming shrubs)
- Sports where you catch and throw (baseball, softball, volleyball)
- Tennis (doubles)
- Using your manual wheelchair
- Using hand cyclers—also called ergometers
- Walking briskly
- Water aerobics

Vigorous Activities
(I can only say a few words without stopping to catch my breath.)

- Aerobic dance
- Biking faster than 10 miles per hour
- Fast dancing
- Heavy gardening (digging, hoeing)
- Hiking uphill
- Jumping rope
- Martial arts (such as karate)
- Race walking, jogging, or running
- Sports with a lot of running (basketball, hockey, soccer)
- Swimming fast or swimming laps
- Tennis (singles)

so alone and may help to keep you motivated. As always, make sure to ask you doctor's advice before starting an exercise program.

Types of Exercise

Exercise roughly breaks down into three categories: flexibility/stretching, aerobic, and resistance training.

- Flexibility exercises essentially involve stretching. Just about anyone can do stretching to maintain or increase flexibility. This can also be a good way to maintain some activity if you're not yet able to exercise more vigorously. Stretching keeps you moving and can be done even if your mobility is limited.

- Aerobic exercise includes activities that burn calories and build your cardiovascular fitness, such as brisk walking, bike riding, jogging, swimming, or any activity that gets your heart rate up. These activities lower the risk of chronic diseases, such as heart attack, stroke, and diabetes. When combined with dietary changes, cardiovascular exercise can help promote weight loss.

- Resistance training, or anaerobic exercise, includes weight lifting and strength training to build muscle. They tone your body and help convert fat into muscle. As many cancer patients gain fat and lose muscle during treatment, resistance training can be particularly helpful in reversing this process.

Ideally, you should try to incorporate both aerobic exercise and weight training into your routine. Each of these act on your body differently and together produce the greatest beneficial effects. Studies in cancer patients consistently find programs of aerobic exercise and resistance training to be beneficial for cardiopulmonary fitness, muscle strength, body composition, and balance, improved walk time, bone mass, and lean muscle mass. This is important for everyone, but particularly for cancer patients, who easily become deconditioned as a result of the disease and its treatment.

Exercise is possible no matter what your physical abilities. It's possible even for those who are bedridden. There are also various fitness classes you can attend, including options for those with physical limitations. Chair aerobics, for instance, is designed for people recovering from medical treatment or those with physical restrictions or limited mobility. It helps to decrease breathlessness and fatigue, improve muscle tone and flexibility, and increase endurance for everyday activities. Other classes may focus on particular goals, such as helping to strengthen bones and maintain bone density in older people or those at risk for osteoporosis. Such programs generally focus on mechanical stresses, including walking, aerobics, balance, and weight training.

Popular among the general population and beneficial for relatively mobile cancer patients are Zumba and Pilates.

- **Zumba** involves Latin-inspired dance moves to the beat of popular music, creating a vigorous aerobic exercise program. It helps to stretch and strengthen core muscles and to help firm the abs, all while burning calories. Most importantly, it's a fun and exhilarating way to work out if you like to dance.

- **Pilates** is a routine of exercise techniques that use balls, resistance bands, and weights. It increases strength, flexibility, endurance, and core stability, while promoting proper use of abdominal muscles to reduce back pain and stress.

Body—and Mind

There are also several Eastern modalities that combine physical activity with mind-body healing.

- **Yoga** originated in ancient India and involves a series of movements, postures, and breath work that is relaxing and can enhance balance, stamina, and range of motion. It contributes to stress relief and promotes general well-being, making it a valuable complementary therapy for cancer patients at any stage of treatment. The word *yoga* means *union* in Sanskrit, an ancient Indian language, suggestive of yoga's role in unifying body, mind, and spirit.

    Yoga is commonly used as a complementary therapy for heart disease, asthma, diabetes, drug addiction, HIV/AIDS, migraine headaches, cancer, and arthritis, among others. Renowned cardiologist Dean Ornish incorporates yoga into his diet and exercise-based program to reverse heart disease. Yoga in fact comes in many forms, the most common of which (at least in the Western world) is Hatha yoga. It can be practiced in a group or individually.

Hatha yoga emphasizes three components: proper breathing, movement, and posture. It involves a series of body postures. While holding various postures, you pay special attention to your breathing, inhaling and exhaling at specific points. You breathe deeply and from the diaphragm. Other special breathing techniques, for example, may involve inhaling through one nostril and out the other. Such breathing is thought to promote relaxation, help to maintain the postures, and to cultivate life energy called prana (similar to the ancient Chinese concept of Qi).

Yoga has been studied in many trials, primarily in women with breast cancer. A recent meta-analysis that pooled data from 10 randomized controlled trials, covering 762 participants, found that yoga can significantly improve anxiety, depression, and stress, among other psychological health factors.[8]

It's not yet clear, however, whether such benefits arise more from the mental (meditation) or physical components of yoga. Although the psychological benefits of yoga are relatively well established, not much evidence has emerged in support of more physical benefits in relation to body composition, fitness, and strength. Consider combining yoga with aerobic exercise and resistance training in order to achieve the greatest benefits for both mind and body.

The best way to start practicing yoga is by taking a class. Finding a good teacher, one who has experience training cancer patients, is key. A typical class lasts from 20 minutes to an hour. It begins with warm-up poses and breathing exercises, followed by a series of postures. Each posture is held for a period of time, usually from 30 seconds to a few minutes. There may then be a period of meditation or rest at the end. It is important to practice yoga regularly in order to achieve the benefits. It's also important to note that, as with any exercise program, some aspects of yoga may be stressful or problematic for you depending on your particular health conditions. Your physician can help you determine whether yoga is appropriate or if there are any specific cautions you should bear in mind.

David, age 45 with leukemia, after starting yoga classes

"I feel like I will once again be strong in my body."

Qigong and **Tai Chi** both originated in China. They are suitable for any age or fitness level and are useful for improving balance, strengthening the body, and clearing the mind. Tai Chi is regularly practiced across modern China by large swaths of the population, including the elderly.

- **Qigong** is an ancient practice that originated around 5,000 years ago. It is a gentle technique that involves various combinations of controlled breathing and simple repetitive motions. It was developed in early China as a means of manipulating the body's vital energy, called Qi or Chi (pronounced "chee"), in order to maintain health and well-being. Although neither the existence of Qi nor the ability to manipulate its flow is supported by modern medical science, Qigong calms the mind, reduces stress and anxiety, and instills a sense of harmony and balance. In the process, it can improve your fitness, balance, and flexibility. Some practitioners experience improved sleep as well. You can learn the practice by taking an in-person class or on your own through DVDs, printed training materials, or online tutorials.

- **Tai Chi** is a newer practice that, like Qigong, combines movement, meditation, and breathing. It likely originated as an exercise to maintain the agility of feudal warriors, but today it has evolved into a daily exercise regimen practiced by the old and young alike, whether sick or well. Tai Chi can be practiced by people of any size or athletic ability and requires neither great strength nor flexibility. It emphasizes concentration, careful attention to breathing, and deliberate, slow motions.

Tai Chi has been extensively studied, and hundreds of publications in the medical literature support various benefits, such as improved balance, reduced risk of falls among the elderly, increased flexibility, and reduced stress, heart rate, and blood pressure. A large review by scientists at Tufts University and the U.S. Institute for Clinical Research and Health Policy Studies, for example, pooled data from more than 40 studies and 3,817 subjects. It found that regular Tai Chi practice reduced stress, anxiety, depression, and mood disturbance and increased self-esteem.[9]

Other analyses have found that Tai Chi may lower blood pressure, with at least one meta-analysis concluding that Tai Chi may be useful as a non-pharmacologic means of managing high blood pressure.

Widely practiced in China for centuries, this exercise technique is becoming increasingly popular in the United States and other Western countries. Tai Chi is a more physically active form of Qigong and is a bit more challenging to learn, but it is an excellent form of gentle exercise. The best way to start is by taking a class—it is offered locally at health clubs, schools, community centers, and other facilities. Some programs are focused more on either the spiritual or fitness aspects of the technique. Books, DVDs, and online tutorials also provide Tai Chi instruction.

Tips for Incorporating Exercise into Your Life

Your goal should be to maintain physical activity as much as possible on an ongoing basis, through treatment and beyond. It's best to exercise in sessions lasting at least 10 minutes at a time and spread out over the course of the week. Unless you were already very active before diagnosis, it may not be reasonable to achieve this level of exercise right away. Don't worry—you can start gradually and build up. You might begin with short walks at a leisurely pace. It's best to set small but achievable goals for yourself along the way.

As always, make sure to ask for your doctor's advice. The degree to which you can be physically active and the specific types of exercise you can engage in will vary depending on your physical condition, the nature of your disease and treatment, and other factors. If you're already on an exercise program, for example, you may need to reduce its intensity during the course of chemotherapy or radiation treatment. As beneficial as exercise can be, it is possible to overdo it, and there are special precautions for those with anemia, bone density issues, or other conditions.

A Few Precautions

The American Cancer Society offers a few precautions in its *Nutrition and Physical Activity Guidelines for Cancer Survivors*, 2012.

Anemia. Avoid exercise beyond activities of daily living until anemia is improved.

Compromised immunity. Avoid public gyms or pools until white blood cell levels improve, to decrease the risk of serious infections.

Severe fatigue. Try just 10 minutes of light exercise daily until you are able to do more.

Radiation treatments. Avoid chlorinated swimming pools, since chlorine can irritate areas of your skin that were irradiated.

Catheters or feeding tubes. Reduce or avoid exposure to pool, lake, or ocean water to minimize the risk of infections at the site where tubes enter your body. Also be cautious if engaging in resistance training, so as not to dislodge catheters.

Other conditions/diseases as well as cancer. Ask your oncologist to determine if these warrant changes to your exercise habits.

Peripheral neuropathy may make it difficult to use affected limbs. If running on a treadmill is challenging, for instance, a stationary bicycle may be a more appropriate option.

Try to find an activity you find fun, whether it is walking, jogging, swimming, gardening, or something else entirely. It will be much easier to exercise regularly if you're doing something that is enjoyable rather than a chore. It may be helpful to exercise in a group setting, such as an exercise class, or with the supervision of a professional. Or if you have a friend who is also trying to become more fit, consider working out with him or her. Having someone else around who shares your goals can often help to keep you motivated. Whatever you do, don't get discouraged! Any physical activity is better than no physical activity. You don't have to run a marathon to experience the benefits.

In fact, you don't necessarily need to join a gym, or even leave your house. Simple changes to your routine, such as taking the stairs instead of the elevator, can make a difference and are good ways to get started. You can also make a point of getting up, stretching, and taking short walks throughout the day. Some people find that measuring the number of steps they take in a day with a pedometer can help motivate them to increase their activity. Pedometers are widely available and relatively inexpensive. Some models can interface with your computer or smart phone and chart your improvement over time.

Studies show that fewer than 10 percent of cancer patients are physically active during treatment, but you can buck that trend! There's no question that lifestyle changes are hard at any point in life, and particularly challenging when you are facing cancer. But the benefits are huge, and they are right there for the taking. Getting in the habit of exercising will make all the difference for your health and well-being.

Notes
1. Moore SC, Patel AV, Matthews CE, Berrington de Gonzalez A, et al. Leisure time physical activity of moderate to vigorous intensity and mortality: a large pooled cohort analysis. *PLoS Med*. 2012;9(11).
2. Irwin ML, Smith AW, McTiernan A, Ballard-Barbash R, et al. Influence of pre- and postdiagnosis physical activity on mortality in breast cancer survivors: the health, eating, activity, and lifestyle study. *J Clin Oncol*. 2008 August 20;26(24):3958–64.

3. Ellsworth RE, Valente AL, Shriver CD, Bittman B, Ellsworth DL. Impact of lifestyle factors on prognosis among breast cancer survivors in the USA. *Expert Rev Pharmacoecon Outcomes Res.* 2012 Aug;12(4):451–64.

4. Hede K. Doctors seek to prevent breast cancer recurrence by lowering insulin levels. *J Natl Cancer Inst.* 2008 Apr 16;100(8):530–2.

5. Mozaffarian D, Hao T, Rimm EB, Willett WC, Hu FB. Changes in diet and lifestyle and long-term weight gain in women and men. *N Engl J Med.* 2011 Jun 23;364(25):2392–404.

6. He C, Bassik MC, Moresi V, Sun K, et al. Exercise-induced BCL2-regulated autophagy is required for muscle glucose homeostasis. *Nature.* 2012 Jan 18;481(7382):511–5.

7. Mikus CR, Oberlin DJ, Libla JL, Taylor AM, Booth FW, Thyfault JP. Lowering physical activity impairs glycemic control in healthy volunteers. *Med Sci Sports Exerc.* 2012 Feb;44(2):225–31.

8. Lin KY, Hu YT, Chang KJ, Lin HF, Tsauo JY. Effects of yoga on psychological health, quality of life, and physical health of patients with cancer: a meta-analysis. *Evid Based Complement Alternat Med.* March, 2011.

9. Wang C, Bannuru R, Ramel J, Kupelnick B, Scott T, Schmid CH. Tai Chi on psychological well-being: systematic review and meta-analysis. *BMC Complement Altern Med.* 2010 May 21.

Worksheet 2: My Weekly Exercise Log

Use this worksheet each week to record any exercise or activities in which you take part. Remember, the U.S. Department of Health and Human Services recommends that you engage in moderate-intensity exercise for 150 minutes or vigorous-intensity exercise for 75 minutes each week (or an equivalent combination of the two). Keeping track of how much you exercise is the first step toward becoming more physically active!

If you have any questions regarding a particular exercise and your condition, be sure to check with your healthcare provider before beginning.

Date	Type of Exercise	For How Long	How It Made Me Feel

Visit www.sprypubcancer.com to download a printable sheet.

Acupuncture

Acupuncture is a safe, painless, and effective modality originally from traditional Chinese medicine. It is an example of a complementary therapy that has made the jump into the mainstream (or at least to the cusp of the mainstream). It has been extensively studied using the tools of modern science, and its value in the management of pain and other conditions has been documented in many randomized clinical trials—the gold standard for medical research. With regard to cancer care, research demonstrates that acupuncture can safely and significantly reduce physical and emotional symptoms associated with cancer and its treatment. Specifically, acupuncture helps to reduce pain, anxiety, and depression, as well as chemotherapy-related and postoperative nausea and vomiting. It may also be useful against hot flashes, xerostomia (extreme dry mouth), chronic fatigue, lymphedema (swelling of the arm following breast cancer surgery involving arm pit lymph nodes), and peripheral neuropathy (nerve-related tingling or lack of feeling in hands or feet).

You should be aware that some misguided acupuncturists claim to treat cancer with acupuncture—a false and incorrect notion. Well-trained, honest acupuncturists know better.

Key Reasons to Consider Acupuncture

- Effectively relieves pain and other symptoms
- May help when conventional pain therapies do not
- Virtually no side effects
- Essentially painless and inexpensive

What Is Involved and How Does Acupuncture Work?

Acupuncture was developed originally in China more than 2,000 years ago. It involves the placement of needles at specific points on the body. These needles are sterile, used only once and then disposed. They are also far thinner than the hollow needles used for injections; acupuncture needles are about the width of a human hair. A skilled acupuncturist inserts these needles just deeply enough to prevent them from falling out. After a needle is placed, the acupuncturist may physically manipulate the needle by twisting it, or may apply heat or a very low electrical current to provide additional stimulation of the acupuncture point. Although it sounds like it might be, acupuncture is not painful.

According to traditional Chinese medicine, vital energy

called Qi or Chi flows throughout the body along channels called meridians. Blockages in this energy flow were thought to cause disease. Needles are placed at specific points, called acupoints, along the body's meridians, which were conceived as channels through which the life energy flows. Illness, it was thought, occurred because of a blockage impeding free flow throughout the meridian.

The needles were thought to unblock the flow, thereby restoring health. Each meridian was believed to be connected to a particular organ system or area of the body, so stimulating acupoints along a particular meridian was thought to treat a problem in a distant part of the body. More than 1,000 acupoints are recognized in modern acupuncture, but most treatment sessions involve the placement of only 10 or 12 needles, which are then left in place for about a half-hour.

Research over recent decades has upheld acupuncture's therapeutic value and provided a more modern understanding of how it actually works. According to modern research, acupuncture is understood to exert its effects by modulating the nervous system and probably also by other physiologic mechanisms currently under study. Brain imaging studies using functional magnetic resonance imaging (fMRI) show that acupuncture activates brain regions that align with the treatment goal. However, much remains to be learned about why acupuncture is so effective at controlling many different symptoms. The existence of meridians is not proven, and there is no scientific evidence to support the ancient concept of a vital life force (Chi). That said, acupuncture works for many people. If it works for you, if it reduces pain or brings back the ability to swallow in patients whose salivary glands were all but destroyed by successful treatment for head and neck cancer, if it has any of the other many good results, it makes little difference that researchers cannot find Chi.

Ron, age 58 with multiple myeloma

"The acupuncture made me sleep like a baby and I believe it has really helped me tolerate lying in a hospital bed for so many days."

A Caution

Acupuncture is used and has been found effective for relieving a variety of conditions and symptoms including arthritis, menstrual symptoms, and chronic pain, and can help to promote smoking cessation and weight loss. It also helps address physical and emotional symptoms of cancer and its treatment. It does this with virtually no side effects. But there is no evidence that it alone can cure cancer or any other disease. Acupuncture is highly valuable as a complementary therapy, but should not be used in place of conventional medical care.

Where Can I Get Acupuncture?

Acupuncture is available at many mainstream hospitals, clinics, and cancer centers, as well as through private acupuncturists. There are more than 15,000 acupuncture practitioners in the United States today. There is a growing group of MDs and doctors of osteopathic medicine (DO) who are also trained to practice acupuncture. Qualified acupuncturists can be found through the National Certification Commission for Acupuncture and Oriental Medicine (NCCAOM) in Washington, D.C. (www.NCCAOM.org). This nonprofit organization was founded to promote safety and competence standards in the practice of oriental medicine. Be sure to find a practitioner who is specifically trained to care for cancer patients.

The Integrative Medicine Department at Memorial Sloan-Kettering Cancer Center offers online Continuing Medical Education classes for healthcare professionals. To request a patient referral for a professional acupuncturist who has successfully completed one of these programs, please contact integmedtraining@mskcc.org.

Mind-Body Therapies

The idea that our thoughts and emotions can influence our physical health is a fundamental belief, passed down since ancient times. It was an element of ancient Greek medicine and virtually all other early healing systems and remains a component of the traditional Chinese medicine and Ayurvedic medicine paradigms still practiced today. The concept has even made its way into our sayings, such as "you'll worry yourself sick" or "you'll give yourself a heart attack." As Western medicine evolved into its modern form, however, mind and body began to be considered as distinct spheres. Mental conditions were studied and treated independent of physical conditions, and vice-versa.

Many diseases once considered having mental or emotional causes are now known to be caused by physical factors, such as bacteria, viruses, or even genetic mutations.

Take gastric ulcers, for example. Once believed to be caused by a stress-induced overproduction of gastric acid, we now know that most ulcers can be attributed to bacteria called *Helicobacter pylori*, which can be eliminated with antibiotics. The mind-body connection has been studied extensively in recent years, and the consensus is that stress, worry, and other mental states do not cause diseases such as cancer. But state of mind can nevertheless affect the experience and progression of many illnesses, among them heart disease, chronic pain, diabetes, arthritis, asthma, and skin problems.

The mind can affect the body in profound ways. There is no better illustration of this than the placebo effect, the phenomenon in which healing occurs simply because the patient expects it to. In fact, years ago doctors frequently gave their patients sugar pills when no effective medicine existed. And, backed by the patients' expectations and trust in their doctor, these placebos often made the patient feel better. Similarly, when studying new hypertension drugs, doctors were initially surprised to find that patients who came in for follow-up visits often had higher blood pressure than they did previously. The stress associated with visiting the doctor had caused a spike in blood pressure, now known as "white-coat hypertension."

The tools of mind-body medicine, such as meditation, guided imagery, and biofeedback, can reduce stress, depression, anxiety, and other negative thoughts and feelings. In so doing, they can help to prevent serious illnesses from worsening, or at least help you through the disease with as little mental and physical wear and tear as possible. Through practice and discipline, mind-body approaches increase your ability to manage stress.

Training the Mind

Mind-body medicine is based on the reciprocal relationship between thoughts/emotions and our physical state. As such, harnessing the connection to achieve greater health can be accomplished from two angles: by training either the mind or the body. We'll provide an overview of mind-based approaches first, and then body-based approaches in the next section.

- Meditation. Focusing your attention—on breathing, an object, or an image—over a period of time. It teaches us to calm our minds and be more present and centered. It can powerfully reduce stress, anxiety, and depression, and can even alleviate pain and other symptoms. Meditation comes in many different forms, but the meditator generally sits still in a quiet environment and practices mental exercises. The meditator is relaxed, yet alert, and focuses on a word, a sound, or even on his or her own breathing. Multiple studies, both recent and going back three decades, show that meditation can lower blood pressure, slow heart rate, reduce stress, and lessen chronic pain.[1]

- Self-hypnosis is easily taught and can be used anytime to reduce anxiety and pain, to make it easier to fall and stay asleep, and improve digestion, among other benefits. It can also be used to help eliminate negative habits such as smoking or weight gain. Most people can be hypnotized, as long as you are receptive to the idea of it. Essentially, hypnosis puts you in a state of focused attention or altered consciousness, in which distractions are blocked out. In this state, you can concentrate on a particular subject, sensation, or problem. Many cancer patients learn the technique and use it to calm their bodies and minds. It can be particularly useful for managing presurgical anxiety and postoperative pain, and can even decrease the need for pain medications.

- **Biofeedback** can help you gain control over how your body responds to stress. It involves the use of a machine to monitor bodily functions such as heart rate, muscle tension, pulse, and breathing rate. All of this information is visible or audible to you in real time. By becoming conscious of how your mental state affects your body's rhythms, you can learn to regulate those responses. This may sound implausible, but with practice it is quite achievable. In a typical biofeedback session, the patient is first connected to monitoring equipment. A biofeedback therapist helps to interpret signals from the machine and walks the patient through mental and physical exercises. Through repetition and practice, the patient learns

Meditation Guide

In case you have never tried meditation, here is a 10-step beginner's guide.

Sit tall. The most common meditation position is sitting. Find a comfortable sitting position and then imagine a string attached to the top of your head pulling your back, neck, and head upward. Sit tall.

Relax your body. Close your eyes and beginning at your feet, consciously think about relaxing each body part moving upward from your feet. Don't forget your shoulders, neck, jaw, face, tongue, and eyes as these are all areas that hold tension.

Be still and silent. Be aware of the sounds around you, but don't react.

Breathe. Turn your attention to your breath, breathing in and out silently and deeply.

Establish a mantra. Your mantra will be a sound, word, or phrase that can be repeated throughout your meditation. It can be spoken aloud our simply repeated to yourself.

Calm your mind. As you focus on your breath or mantra, allow your mind to become calm. As thoughts come to you, don't dwell on them. Simply acknowledge them and set them aside, returning to thinking about your breathing or mantra.

Your meditation time. When beginning, you may want to meditate for a shorter time period (5 or 10 minutes) and extend it as you become more comfortable. Some people like to set timers or count a number of breaths.

Ending your meditation. Bring your conscious attention back to your surroundings. Acknowledge your presence in the space around you. Gently move your fingers and toes, moving to your hands and feet, and then arms and legs. Take your time in getting up.

Practice often. Short periods of regular meditation have more positive effects than a single weekly meditation period.

Practice everywhere. Often beginners are most comfortable in a quiet place at home, but as you become more practiced at meditation try expanding your practice locations. Including natural settings and even work locations can be an excellent stress reliever.

Try meditation today to benefit from the calming of your mind and the relaxing of your body.

how to harness his or her thoughts, breathing, and posture to achieve the desired results, such as reducing anxiety. Not everyone is interested in biofeedback or comfort-

Memorial Sloan-Kettering Cancer Center offers a number of free videos on integrative medicine, including meditation and yoga. Visit www.mskcc.org/cancer-care/integrative-medicine/multimedia.

able using the monitoring equipment. This is only one of many ways to take advantage of the mind-body connection, so try one of the others if this one is not right for you.

Training the Body

There are also several Eastern modalities that approach mind-body healing through physical activity.

- **Yoga** involves a series of movements, postures, and breath work that is helpful for improving fitness, stamina, balance, and range of motion. Some types of yoga also use meditation. Yoga contributes to stress relief and promotes general well-being, making it a valuable complementary therapy for cancer patients at any stage of treatment. The word *yoga* means *union* in Sanskrit, an ancient Indian language, which is fitting because its regular practice helps to unify body, mind, and spirit. There are many forms of yoga, but the most common in the Western world is Hatha yoga. It can be practiced in a group, at home with a loved one, or individually.

- **Qigong** and **Tai Chi** both originated in China and help to improve balance, strengthen the body, and clear the mind. They combine movement and meditation and are suitable for any age or fitness level. Qigong involves various combinations of controlled breathing and simple repetitive motions. It is a gentle technique that improves stamina, while calming the mind; it can improve sleep and instill a sense of harmony and balance. Tai Chi is a bit more challenging to learn, but is an excellent daily exercise regimen. It involves concentration, careful attention to breathing, and deliberate, slow motions. It has similar benefits to Qigong. If you are interested in these techniques, you may want to try both. Also remember that there are various styles; certain ones may suit you better than others and you can develop your own variations on the theme.

A Caution

Mind-body therapies reduce stress and can improve quality of life. They are inexpensive, can be done on your own, and they do not lead to harmful side effects, but they do not *cure* disease all on their own. However, the mind-body connection is powerful and beneficial. Harnessing your mind to help heal your body and reduce stress can help you achieve the optimal duo of emotional and physical health.

Where Can I Get These Therapies?

Most mind-body therapies, with the exception of biofeed-back, don't require any specialized equipment and can be practiced on your own or in groups, at home or elsewhere. You can learn these techniques through private sessions with a trained therapist, through classes offered at gyms and community centers, among other places, or on your own with the help of DVDs, CDs, or YouTube videos that you can find online (see the link to MSKCC videos earlier in this chapter). More information about hypnosis is available from the American Society of Clinical Hypnosis (www.asch.net/genpubinfo.htm) and other Internet sources. If you are interested in biofeedback, you can find a certified therapist through the Biofeedback Certification International Alliance (www.bcia.org).

Note

1. Reiner K, Tibi L, Lipsitz JD. Do mindfulness-based interventions reduce pain intensity? A critical review of the literature. *Pain Med.* 2013 Feb;14(2):230–42; Kabat-Zinn J, Lipworth L, Burney R. The clinical use of mindfulness meditation for the self-regulation of chronic pain. *J Behav Med.* 1985 Jun;8(2):163–90.

Massage

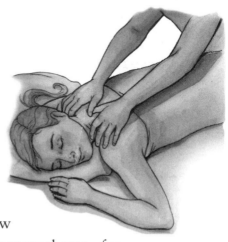

Massage comes in many forms, all of which are well known to relieve stress and to promote relaxation. It is valuable for anyone, but is now commonly used as a complementary therapy for people with various illnesses, including cancer. Hospitals all over the world increasingly offer massage therapy to their patients, and its benefits for pain relief, physical and emotional well-being, and overall quality of life are well established. It can also help with issues that are exacerbated by tight muscles, such as insomnia, headache, and backache.

Therapeutic massage dates back several millennia. *The Yellow Emperor's Classic of Internal Medicine*, a Chinese medical text published in 2700 B.C., specifies that "breathing exercises, massage of the skin and flesh, and exercises of the hand and feet" be used to treat paralysis, chills, and fever. Massage is even depicted in early Egyptian tomb paintings.

Swedish massage, the most popular form used today in the United States, focuses on relaxing the muscles and soft tissues through gentle physical manipulation. Eastern types of massage, such as Shiatsu and Reiki, focus more on restoring the body's energy and tend to be gentler. While the underlying philosophy differs, the ultimate effects are much the same. Both complement the body's natural healing ability, promoting relaxation and stress relief, while helping the body to recover from physical injury and emotional strain.

Massage therapy typically is provided in a room with a sheet-covered massage table. The room usually is dimly lit, with soothing background music. The specific massage techniques used vary based on your preferences and those of the practitioner, so be sure to tell your therapist what you expect and are comfortable with. Most sessions last from 30 minutes to one hour.

Massage Therapy for Cancer Patients

It is important to use a licensed massage therapist who also was trained and certified to work with cancer patients.

Several variations of massage therapy are worth mentioning here:

- **Aromatherapy massage** involves the use of aromatic plant extracts and essential oils. It can improve mood, restore balance throughout the body, and promote general well-being. Some patients prefer massage therapy without aromatherapy as they find it nauseating; others enjoy the aroma.

- **Reiki** is a form of very light touch massage. It promotes physical and emotional well-being and deep relaxation, and is especially useful for hospitalized or weak individuals.
- **Shiatsu** is a form of Japanese massage that uses hand pressure and stretching to promote balance in body and mind. Shiatsu may be performed either on the floor or on a massage table, depending on patient preference and what is appropriate given the clinical status of the individual. Patients receiving such treatment are fully clothed.
- **Swedish massage** involves therapeutic manipulation of the muscles using hand movements. It relieves muscular tension, stimulates circulation, and aids in relaxation.

Linda, age 54 with rectum/colon cancer, following massage therapy

"I was in excruciating pain from the radiation treatments. Agonizing. When I came in I could barely walk. Nothing helped me with the pain like lying on the table and having your kind hands help me to relax. I can't thank you enough."

Reflexology

Strictly speaking, reflexology is not massage (though it does feel that way when you receive it!). It is an ancient practice of applying pressure to specific parts of the hands, feet, and/or ears. Foot reflexology is most common today. The foot is used as a map of the entire body; pressing specific areas of the foot is believed to heal problems in the corresponding part of the body. Most foot reflexology is based on the work of an American nurse and physical therapist in the 1930s named Eunice Ingham. She developed detailed maps of the feet and through trial and error showed that pressing the arch of the foot, for example, affects the inner organs. The technique is very relaxing, reduces stress, relieves pain, and increases circulation. It can also help with some chronic problems, such as headaches, asthma, or bowel issues, but it cannot (and does not claim to) cure any illness. It is especially helpful for very ill patients who cannot easily tolerate even gentle body massage therapy.

Although you or a family member theoretically can learn the foot massage techniques and apply them, foot reflexology is typically performed by a trained reflexologist. The patient lies on a massage table while the reflexologist gently massages each foot and then applies pressure to the various reflex points. Such treatments typically last from 30 minutes to one hour. Although the beliefs on which reflexology is based—that

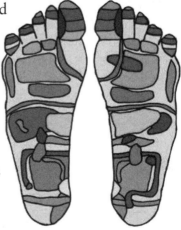

manipulating specific points on the foot can affect distant organ systems—is not necessarily valid, foot reflexology is safe, relaxing, and inexpensive. If nothing else, it is worthwhile as a very pleasant foot massage.

A Caution

Massage can be extraordinarily valuable for relaxation and to help relieve stress, muscle tension, and various associated problems. But as with other complementary therapies, it does not treat or *cure* disease. Be sure to seek a massage therapist who is specifically trained to work with cancer patients.

Although massage is very safe, you should avoid it if you have fever, acute inflammation, infection, phlebitis, thrombosis, or jaundice. Furthermore, you should not be massaged near the site of a recent injury, to avoid exacerbating it, and of course all areas of the body containing ports, bandaged surgical sites, and the like are to be avoided.

Where Can I Get Massage Therapy?

There are many organizations that provide information about massage therapy and can help you find a qualified therapist locally. Among them are the International Massage Association (www.imagroup.com), the American Massage Therapy Association (www.amtamassage.org), and the U.S. National Certification Board for Therapeutic Massage and Bodywork (www.ncbtmb.org). The International Institute of Reflexology (www.reflexology-uk.net) provides further information on reflexology and can help you find a reflexologist in your area.

> The Integrative Medicine Department at Memorial Sloan-Kettering Cancer Center offers online Continuing Medical Education classes for healthcare professionals. To request a patient referral for a massage therapist who has successfully completed one of these programs, please contact integmedtraining@mskcc.org.

Creative Therapies

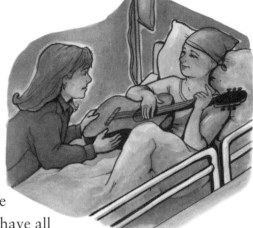

Creativity is inherently therapeutic, whether creating something ourselves or enjoying the creativity of others. We have all experienced the joy of viewing or creating artwork, playing or listening to music, hearing or telling a good joke or funny story. Seeking joy through creativity is not only fun, it can also promote healing.

Creative therapies include art, music, dance, and humor. They all engage the senses and involve either producing or experiencing a work of art. In so doing, they can decrease stress and anxiety, promote relaxation, and entertain patients with serious illnesses. They can also relieve pain and discomfort by redirecting your attention and provide a healthy way, usually without words, to express fears and feelings about your disease or discomfort. To be clear, these creative modalities are all complementary therapies to be used along with conventional treatment; none can cure disease in and of itself.

These types of therapies are generally inexpensive and produce health benefits without the risk of side effects. You can practice them independently or they can be facilitated by a professional therapist. Many hospitals offer creative therapies to patients while they are hospitalized and may even send professional therapists to patient rooms. Practitioners frequently start off as artists themselves, and then become interested in the medical application of their art.

Some creative outlets routinely used are:

- **Art therapy** allows patients to freely create through drawing, painting, or even sculpture and to express themselves without fear of judgment or criticism. The creative process helps promote self-awareness, as well as physical and emotional healing, while also building self-esteem. Sometimes it can be very difficult to verbalize our thoughts, fears, and other hidden emotions. In these cases, expressing them through artwork can be therapeutic. Art therapists provide advice, emotional support, and the paintbrush and paper—or whatever tools are needed.
- **Music therapy** harnesses the power of music to uplift our moods and arouse our emotions. It involves performing, creating, or listening to music to encourage healing and promote a general sense of well-being. Patients listen to or perform music with the guidance

of a professional music therapist. The therapist can help to develop lyrics, improvise with the patient, or simply provide technical and emotional support. The practice can enhance relaxation, creativity, pleasure, and self-expression while helping to reduce pain and feelings of isolation. Music therapy is provided by musicians who received training, typically graduate training, in the use of music (rather than only words) as therapy. It is especially helpful in a hospital setting.

- **Dance therapy** is a multisensory approach that combines movement, music, and social interaction. It supports patients in expressing the experience of their illness and helps to reduce feelings of isolation by promoting relationships with others. It also provides excellent physical exercise, with benefits to muscle strength, balance, and overall fitness. Dance therapy provides an outlet for expressing feelings and releasing tension through movement. It can be relaxing, exhilarating, and empowering and can be effective regardless of your age or physical ability.

- **Humor therapy** is the purposeful use of humor as a complementary therapy to enliven and enhance well-being for people who are ill. Laughter, funny as it may sound, can actually make a big difference. It improves quality of life, redirects attention away from chronic pain, and encourages relaxation and stress release. Many hospitals provide humorous books or videos, or even trained laughter therapists. Humor can also provide a means for communicating with caregivers and loved ones and can be an effective icebreaker when thoughts or feelings are difficult to express. As an old Irish saying goes "a good laugh and a long sleep are the best cures in the doctor's book."

> **Paul, age 45 with sarcoma of the thigh, following music therapy**
>
> "That was so beautiful, so spiritual. I could see myself rising above this pain." The intervention was vocal toning/vocal holding technique employed to induce relaxation and decrease perception of pain.

Where Can I Get Creative Therapies?

Many hospitals have art, music, and/or dance therapists on staff and offer these services to hospitalized patients. Professional therapists often come to patient rooms. Other medical centers have recreation areas where music, art, or dance can be informally performed, and humor can be practiced just about anywhere. On an outpatient basis, these creative arts can be performed on your own, with family or friends, or with the help of a private therapist.

Part Three

Symptom Relief with Complementary Therapies

More from Paul's brother, age 45 with sarcoma of the thigh, following music therapy

"… During the [Music Therapy session], the focus was less on my brother's 'condition' than the making of the music. First, they would choose a song to play, then [the music therapist] would learn it on the guitar, then they would record it together on mini-disc. Their recording sessions were full of laughter but were also intensely serious. When the disc player was running, my brother wasn't in a hospital, he was in a recording studio; he wasn't infirm, he was full of health and vigor. He wasn't unfree, he was free."

Among the most common symptoms of cancer and its treatment are pain, depression, and fatigue. All too frequently, patients do not feel that such symptoms are best, or even adequately, managed by conventional approaches alone. Various complementary therapies can help. Sometimes, a single modality, such as acupuncture, for example, may do the trick. More often, a combination of approaches, integrating multiple complementary and/or conventional therapies, may provide the most effective relief.

The purpose of this section is to serve as a reference guide to complementary therapies organized by symptom type. You need not read through it in its entirety. Simply look up the symptoms that are relevant to you, although the therapies discussed are not all-inclusive. Just because a particular approach is not mentioned does not necessarily mean it isn't helpful. Our goal is to provide you with an overview of the strongest evidence, and to guide you as you begin to explore complementary options that are both effective and safe.

Symptoms Often Associated with Surgery, Chemotherapy, and Other Cancer Treatments

Pain
Fatigue
Anxiety, stress, and depression
Nausea and vomiting
Hot flashes
Sexual problems
Xerostomia (extreme dry mouth)
Lymphedema
Neuropathy

Some complementary therapies have been extensively studied; others have less research behind them. In this section, we focus primarily on those that have been proven safe and either effective or probably so. Always discuss any complementary therapies you are interested in with your doctor before starting them, to ensure there will be no negative interactions with your other treatments. This is particularly important for herbs and dietary supplements, which generally should be avoided during cancer treatment.

Managing Pain

Cancer patients almost always contend with pain in some form—whether from the tumor itself or as a side effect of treatment. Complementary therapies such as acupuncture, massage therapy, mind-body techniques, and music therapy can help reduce this pain safely and without toxicity or side effects. These therapies can be particularly effective in conjunction with conventional pain medications, boosting the results and potentially decreasing the amount of prescription drugs required to keep you comfortable. They may also be helpful on their own, in cases where medication either isn't effective or causes intolerable side effects. Patients who require long-term pain management may also develop a tolerance to pain medications, making complementary therapies an attractive alternative for getting relief without side effects or drug dependence. For these reasons, patients with chronic pain tend to be heavy users of complementary therapies.

Managing Pain with Acupuncture

Acupuncture is widely used for pain in the general population—both acute pain, such as associated with a dental
procedure, and chronic pain, such as headache. Increasingly,
acupuncture is used for cancer-related pain, too, as a growing
number of studies find it to be effective. Acupuncture appears
to work by stimulating the nervous system, causing the
release of certain chemicals in the brain that control pain.
Brain imaging studies suggest that it can deactivate areas of
the brain involved in pain perception.

One of the first well-designed trials of acupuncture for
chronic cancer pain was conducted in 2003. It tested auricular acupuncture—in which needles are placed at acupoints
on the ear—for patients whose pain remained despite ongoing treatment with pain medication. Patients were needled
either at the correct acupressure points or at non-acupressure
points on their ears. A third group had pressure (as opposed
to needles) applied at non-acupuncture points. After two
months of these treatments, pain intensity had decreased by
36 percent in the patients who received correct acupuncture.
Little difference was observed in the two control groups,
showing not only that acupuncture was effective, but also
that the specific points mattered. Needling random points did
not have the same effect as proper acupuncture.[1]

Another study, conducted at Memorial Sloan-Kettering
Cancer Center, tested acupuncture specifically in patients
with cancer of the head or neck who had received neck

dissection surgery. Patients either received acupuncture weekly for four weeks, or usual care from their physician. Those in the acupuncture group reported significant reductions in pain compared to their usual-care counterparts.[2]

Yet another high-quality study found acupuncture to be effective at reducing joint pain in breast cancer patients taking aromatase inhibitor drugs. Joint pain is a common and unpleasant side effect of such medication, which blocks the production of estrogen. This randomized trial compared true versus sham acupuncture at multiple points on the ears and elsewhere on the body. Women in the acupuncture group had significantly less pain at six weeks.[3]

Not all studies are this unequivocal, but acupuncture clearly is promising as a complementary therapy for alleviating cancer-related pain. Given acupuncture's safety record, it is a good option for pain control without any major downsides. Insertion of acupuncture needles is virtually painless, and most patients actually find the treatments relaxing. It is important, however, that you make sure to choose an acupuncturist who is trained and certified to work with cancer patients.

Katherine speaking about her husband's care

"During February, my husband was an inpatient for his liposarcoma. He was fortunate to receive massage and acupuncture professionals' care. The acupuncture turned out to bring tremendous relief from pain."

Managing Pain with Massage Therapy

Massage therapy may be very beneficial for chronic pain and is widely available in hospital programs. This modality comes in many forms—Swedish massage, foot reflexology, Reiki, and other very gentle-touch massage therapies—and its effects go beyond relieving sore muscles. It is calming and relaxing, improves blood and lymph circulation, reduces stress, and helps with sleep, among other benefits. All of this factors into its ability to reduce pain.

Clinical trials show that massage can diminish pain, anxiety, and other symptoms related to cancer treatment. Although the number of high-quality studies is limited, results confirm that body or foot massage can decrease pain in cancer patients. One study of nearly 1,300 patients showed that massage improved patients' pain scores by 40 percent.[4] In general, most patients feel better after massage therapy, reporting substantial relief of symptoms for hours or sometimes days after treatment.

Furthermore, massage therapy is very safe. The antiquated belief that massage might spread cancer around the body has

---

Barbara, age 63 with lung cancer

"After my surgery, I realize now I was afraid to move, afraid to breathe. It wasn't just the pain ... really even after the pain was gone, I know that there was fear. I really think that the massages allowed me to confront that and try and let it go. I don't know if I would have been able to do that on my own."

long since been proven incorrect. Nevertheless, it's important that you find a therapist trained to work with cancer patients if you seek massage outside of the hospital setting.

Managing Pain with Mind-Body Therapies

Mind-body techniques, such as meditation, self-hypnosis, guided imagery, and yoga, are particularly useful for those who want to take an active role in their own well-being. These approaches essentially teach you how to control your mind and, in turn, your body, to reduce the sense of pain, anxiety, and stress. The idea that pain perception can be influenced by a person's attitudes and beliefs, which can be altered with the help of mind-body therapies, has become increasingly mainstream in recent years. The fact that place-bos work—that belief can affect biology—is essentially proof of concept.

> **Kristen, age 36 with advanced breast cancer**
>
> "After my guided meditation practice, I felt very much at peace, which I feel is pretty remarkable given the current circumstances."

Randomized controlled trials show that self-hypnosis, which essentially helps reprogram the brain's responses to signals from the body, can significantly reduce pain. In one study, patients who received hypnosis training prior to undergoing bone marrow transplant reported significantly less pain than those who did not receive the training.[5]

Similarly, another study found that metastatic breast cancer patients who attended group therapy with hypnosis weekly for one year reported significantly less pain and moodiness than patients who attended weekly group therapy without hypnosis.[6] A National Institutes of Health panel strongly recommends the use of hypnosis for cancer-related pain. Mind-body techniques such as self-hypnosis, guided imagery, and relaxation are easy to learn and can be very beneficial when practiced before and during painful or stressful procedures such as chemotherapy and radiation therapy, and in preparation for surgery.

Music therapy, too, often can reduce pain and anxiety. One large clinical trial found that music therapy after surgery reduced both patients' pain levels and the amount of morphine they needed to remain comfortable.[7]

Family of a patient following her death

" The music that you brought to Mom during her hospital stays gave her some of the most joyful moments she was able to experience in her final weeks, even when she was in terrible pain and distress. We cannot thank you enough for that gift, and for the meaningful time we were able to share as a family while you played and sang to her. Please know that you have our everlasting gratitude for the pleasure you brought to Mom. "

Some herbs and supplements used topically also have pain-reducing properties. Among the more promising are capsaicin, a compound found in chili pepper, and an herb called boswellia. Capsaicin cream is applied to painful areas of the skin and is believed to diminish pain by desensitizing nerve endings. It first causes heat, pain, or a burning sensation when applied, but ultimately brings relief. One study found that use of capsaicin cream over 16 weeks significantly reduced the perception of pain in cancer patients after surgery.[8]

Because capsaicin can be extremely irritating to the mucous membranes and to the eyes, avoid contact with eyes and do not use over irritated or broken skin. Wear gloves when applying to the skin. Do not use if you are on ACE inhibitors, as capsaicin can increase the incidence of cough that is associated with ACE inhibitors. Also, if you are taking sedatives, capsaicin may increase sedation, or if you are taking theophylline or antihypertensives, capsaicin may affect their actions or increase absorption. The problems and precautions associated with capsaicin would not make it a first or even second choice for pain relief.

Notes

1. Alimi D, Rubino C, Pichard-Léandri E, Fermand-Brulé S, Dubreuil-Lemaire ML, Hill C. Analgesic effect of auricular acupuncture for cancer pain: a randomized, blinded, controlled trial. *J Clin Oncol.* 2003 Nov 15;21(22):4120–6.

2. Pfister DG, Cassileth BR, Deng GE, Yeung KS, et al. Acupuncture for pain and dysfunction after neck dissection: results of a randomized controlled trial. *J Clin Oncol.* 2010 May 20;28(15):2565–70.

3. Oh B, Kimble B, Costa DS, Davis E, et al. Acupuncture for treatment of arthralgia secondary to aromatase inhibitor therapy in women with

early breast cancer: pilot study. *Acupunct Med.* 2013 May 30.

4. Cassileth BR, Vickers AJ. Massage therapy for symptom control: outcome study at a major cancer center. *J Pain Symptom Manage.* 2004 Sep;28(3):244–9.

5. Syrjala KL, Cummings C, Donaldson GW. Hypnosis or cognitive behavioral training for the reduction of pain and nausea during cancer treatment: a controlled clinical trial. *Pain.* 1992 Feb;48(2):137–46.

6. Nash MR, Tasso A. The effectiveness of hypnosis in reducing pain and suffering among women with metastatic breast cancer and among women with temporomandibular disorder. *Int J Clin Exp Hypn.* 2010 Oct;58(4):497–504.

7. Good M, Anderson GC, Stanton-Hicks M, Grass JA, Makii M. Relaxation and music reduce pain after gynecologic surgery. *Pain Manag Nurs.* 2002 Jun;3(2):61–70.

8. Ellison N, Loprinzi CL, Kugler J, Hatfield AK, et al. Phase III placebo-controlled trial of capsaicin cream in the management of surgical neuropathic pain in cancer patients. *J Clin Oncol.* 1997 Aug;15(8):2974–80.

Fatigue

Fatigue is a common issue for many cancer patients. It is a persistent sensation of tiredness that is brought on or exacerbated by chemotherapy, radiation treatment, medications, or stress, among other factors. In a survey of cancer patients, 60 percent reported that they experienced fatigue at least once a week during their most recent chemotherapy cycle. Although most patients' energy levels rebound within a few months of finishing treatment, others continue to feel fatigued for an extended period. Moreover, cancer treatment is not the only cause; you may find that you have less energy even before you begin treatment. Being diagnosed with cancer is a difficult and stressful experience in and of itself, as you know only too well, and fatigue can be a product of that.

But don't despair. Fatigue, like many other cancer-related symptoms, can be improved. Exercise, yoga, acupuncture, and massage are among the complementary therapies that can help you to regain your energy. Make sure to discuss your symptoms with your doctor, so he or she can make sure there is no underlying cause that should be corrected medically. For instance, fatigue may be caused by anemia, thyroid problems, or sleep disruption, among other issues, in which case those should be addressed first.

Managing Fatigue with Exercise

It's understandable if you feel too tired to move about or work out, but you may want to reconsider. Although exercise seems tiring, it can actually help combat your fatigue. By putting a little energy in, you can get a lot more out in return. It can be as simple as a period of brisk walking each day, working out in a gym (ideally with the guidance of a trained professional), swimming, or any other activity that is safe for your condition.

In a recent analysis, University of Connecticut researchers pooled the results of 44 separate randomized controlled trials covering more than 3,000 fatigued patients with various types of cancer. Those who exercised experienced higher energy levels and reported significant reductions in their cancer-related fatigue compared to control subjects who did not exercise. This was particularly true for older patients who engaged in moderate-intensity resistance training (strength-building exercises such as lifting weights). Older patients in fact experienced greater reductions in fatigue than younger ones. Furthermore, the more intense the exercise program, the greater the improvements in energy levels.[1]

Similarly, a 2008 review article produced by the well-regarded Cochrane Collaboration examined 28 trials and concluded that cancer-related fatigue was improved significantly more in patients who exercised than in those who did not. This was true for patients both during and after active cancer treatment. Although most of the trials included breast cancer patients, there is no reason to believe that the finding wouldn't apply to those with other cancer diagnoses as well.[2]

Generally, studies suggest that exercise can be safe and effectively reduce fatigue even during chemotherapy and radiation, and for many different cancer types. It appears that even low-intensity exercise—aerobic and/or resistance—can be helpful. Because cancer treatment can lead to muscle wasting, exercise may help to diminish fatigue by building muscle and restoring its function. There are other theories as well, as the exact cause of cancer-related fatigue is not well understood.

Remember that reduced fatigue is only one of the many physical and psychological benefits of exercise, from improved stamina, agility, and muscle tone to heightened self-confidence, self-esteem, and happiness. As discussed earlier, it also may reduce the risk of recurrence and lengthen survival time. All things considered, an exercise program is a great place to start for tackling cancer symptoms such as fatigue and for generally enhancing your health. Its importance cannot be overstressed.

Managing Fatigue with Yoga

By combining physical exercise with meditation, yoga practice promotes relaxation and may help to reduce fatigue
(as well as stress, anxiety, and depression). In yoga, the practitioner maintains various physical postures while focusing
on the body and breathing. Most patients find it to be enjoyable, and perhaps more peaceful than ordinary exercise. It is
sometimes practiced as part of a broader meditation program
called mindfulness-based stress reduction.

To date, very few trials of yoga or other lifestyle changes
have specifically targeted cancer patients with persistent
fatigue. The studies that do exist are small but encouraging.

In a recent randomized controlled trial conducted at the
University of California–Los Angeles, researchers sought to
determine the effectiveness of yoga for breast cancer patients
with persistent fatigue. The study included 31 women who
had completed cancer treatments at least 6 months before
and who had no other medical conditions that would explain
their fatigue. Half of the women completed a 12-week yoga
program (specially designed for fatigued patients) and the
other half a 12-week health education program. The patients
who practiced yoga saw a significant decline in their fatigue
and a significant increase in vigor compared to others in
the health education class. Moreover, the benefits lasted for
at least 3 months after the program ended. Despite their
fatigue, 80 percent of the patients attended at least 20 of the
24 yoga classes offered, suggesting that they found the

experience to be worthwhile, rewarding, and pleasant.[3]

The suggestion that yoga may help cancer patients to overcome persistent fatigue is quite promising, although there hasn't been enough research yet to prove these effects. There is, however, a body of evidence that shows that yoga can significantly decrease stress, anxiety, and depression. And decreasing those debilitating problems can indirectly reduce fatigue. Most importantly, yoga is very safe when practiced with the guidance of a professional trained to work with cancer patients. If other methods have not successfully reduced your fatigue or if you are interested in yoga for other reasons, it is worth a try.

Managing Fatigue with Acupuncture

Although acupuncture's benefits are most well documented for pain and nausea, many studies suggest that acupuncture may also help to alleviate cancer-related fatigue.

One notable trial compared the effects of acupuncture, self-acupressure, and sham (fake) acupressure on fatigued cancer patients who had previously completed chemotherapy and found that both acupuncture and acupressure significantly improved fatigue. Acupressure is like acupuncture except that points on the body are stimulated by physical pressure rather than with needles. As such, you can perform acupressure at home on yourself, without the need for an acupuncturist.

In this study, sham acupressure involved pressure at the

wrong points and thus should not work, serving as a control. Patients receiving acupuncture received six 20-minute sessions over 2 weeks, and patients receiving acupressure were taught which points on their body to press/massage and then did so daily for two weeks. Although the study was small, with only 47 participants, the results were remarkable: patients in the acupuncture group experienced a 36 percent improvement in fatigue, compared to 19 percent for the acupressure group, and 0.6 percent for the control, sham acupressure group.[4]

Another small study, conducted by UCLA researchers, assessed the value of acupuncture in women who had completed treatment for breast cancer but suffered from ongoing fatigue. One group of patients received once-weekly acupuncture treatments for 8 weeks combined with a wellness education class. A second group received usual care from their physicians (no acupuncture). Patients in the acupuncture group ultimately experienced a 66 percent reduction in fatigue.[5]

Researchers are still probing the effects of acupuncture on fatigue and further study is ongoing. Given that existing evidence has been largely favorable, however, and that acupuncture is extremely safe, it may be worth considering for your fatigue symptoms. Acupuncture also has many other well-documented benefits such as easing pain. If you choose to get this type of treatment, make sure to seek out an acupuncturist who is trained to work with cancer patients, and tell the acupuncturist about all symptoms you may be experiencing, such as pain and depression as well as fatigue. The acupuncturist should be able to treat all of those problems at the same time.

Other Things That May Help Manage Fatigue

Very limited studies suggest that massage or music therapy also can be beneficial for relieving fatigue, at least in some cases. Similarly, some herbs and dietary supplements, such as ginseng, vitamin B_{12}, and folic acid, may be helpful for increasing energy, but they have not been well studied and results are mixed. Cancer patients should be particularly cautious—it's a good idea to discuss them with your doctor before using any herbs or supplements.

Memorial Sloan-Kettering Cancer Center (MSKCC) has developed a website and a free app containing everything you need to know about herbs and other dietary supplements. Visit MSKCC.org/AboutHerbs for more information or to download the free app. Healthcare providers can also obtain additional information under the "Professionals" tab.

Notes

1. Brown JC, Huedo-Medina TB, Pescatello LS, Pescatello SM, Ferrer RA, Johnson BT, et al. Efficacy of exercise interventions in modulating cancer-related fatigue among adult cancer survivors: a meta-analysis. *Cancer Epidemiol Biomarkers Prev.* 2011 Jan;20(1):123–33.

2. The effect of exercise on fatigue associated with cancer. *Cochrane Database Syst Rev: Plain Lang Summaries*. November 14, 2012. http://www.ncbi.nlm.nih.gov/pubmedhealth/PMH0013760/.

3. Bower JE, Garet D, Sternlieb B, Ganz PA, et al. Yoga for persistent fatigue in breast cancer survivors: a randomized controlled trial. *Cancer*. 2012 Aug 1;118(15):3766–75.

4. Molassiotis A, Sylt P, Diggins H. The management of cancer-related fatigue after chemotherapy with acupuncture and acupressure: a randomised controlled trial. *Complement Ther Med*. 2007 Dec;15(4):228–37.

5. Johnston MF, Hays RD, Subramanian SK, Elashoff RM, et al. Patient education integrated with acupuncture for relief of cancer-related fatigue randomized controlled feasibility study. *BMC Complement Altern Med*. 2011 Jun 25;11:49.

Anxiety, Stress, and Depression

Cancer inevitably stirs up many feelings. It's normal to become anxious or stressed-out, and many patients and family members face feelings of depression. Help, however, is readily available. Talking about your feelings with people you trust can be beneficial. In some cases, medications may help. But there is also a whole realm of complementary therapies for your possible use. Some, like meditation, require some effort on your part, and others, like massage, are completely passive. Many of these therapies may be available through your hospital. Whatever your condition or preferences, something in this realm will likely fit. It's important that you choose what feels right for you.

Managing Anxiety, Stress, and Depression with Mind-Body Therapies

Meditation, in which you focus awareness and attention on your breathing or on some other sound or object, is probably the most popular and widely used mind-body technique. It has been studied extensively over the past few decades and is becoming increasingly mainstream. Regular meditation decreases anxiety, wards off bouts of chronic depression, and helps patients to cope more effectively. Meditation is frequently combined with yoga as part of a program called "mindfulness-based stress reduction" (MBSR). In one study, breast and prostate cancer patients who took an 8-week MBSR course and continued practicing on their own experienced increased quality of life and decreased stress. The patients' blood pressure improved, and stress hormone levels decreased. These benefits lasted for at least 12 months.[1]

Multiple controlled trials involving cancer patients with varying diagnoses and stages of disease show that meditation decreases anxiety and depression.[2]

Jan, age 57 with ovarian cancer

" What I learned about meditation came in handy when I was called to an MRI late last night. When I found out it was an hour in that tube I panicked but then remembered the techniques. I actually meditated to the sounds of the MRI machine, which was quite musical, rhythmic, and beautiful in a weird way. My brain was picking up words, patterns, and layers in the noise and I relaxed and melted into the machine like I did here in the bed. I came out of the MRI more relaxed than I went in, and it was actually an enjoyable experience from the perspective of a unique meditative/spiritual experience and learning something about my ability to control pain and anxiety. "

Meditation, however, is only one of many mind-body therapies that can help to reduce psychological symptoms and control pain. Others include biofeedback, guided imagery, hypnosis, relaxation therapy, and more. All of these approaches are effective strategies that harness the reciprocal relationship between mind and body to produce symptom relief. An analysis of 116 separate studies on this topic concluded that mind-body therapies could benefit cancer patients with anxiety, depression, moodiness, and difficulty coping.[3]

Relaxation therapy, for example, may be as effective as anti-anxiety medication. A randomized controlled trial that compared relaxation therapy with the drug Xanax (alprazolam) found that both significantly reduced anxiety and depression, although the medication was faster-acting and slightly more powerful for depression. Still, relaxation had nearly the same outcome, at lower cost and with no side effects. Hypnosis also reduces anxiety and distress and may be particularly effective in children.

Mind-body therapies are well worth trying out. Select those that appeal to you. The various types of mind-body therapy are described in detail in part two of this book, if you would like to learn more.

Managing Anxiety, Stress, and Depression with Massage Therapy

It is not surprising that massage therapy is very beneficial for stress relief. Several studies show that massage reduces anxiety and related symptoms, probably at least in part by decreasing levels of stress hormones. A study in breast cancer patients found increased levels of serotonin and dopamine and decreased stress hormone levels after massage, with patients reporting reduced anxiety, depression, and anger.[4]

In one small randomized trial, 35 patients received either massage or usual care while waiting to receive bone marrow transplants. After only one week and an average of three massage sessions, patients reported considerably less anxiety. Fatigue, distress, and nausea also were diminished.[5]

A larger study of 87 hospitalized cancer patients tested the effects of foot massage on anxiety. Patients who received foot massage reported significant decreases in their pain and anxiety, compared with patients who did not get the massage.[6] Interestingly, studies suggest that aromatherapy can magnify the effects of massage on anxiety. In aromatherapy massage, aromatic oils are added to the massage oil, adding pleasant aromas to the experience and further promoting relaxation.

Perhaps most importantly, massage is both pleasant and very safe. Make sure to seek out a therapist trained to work with cancer patients; this is particularly important if you are getting massage therapy outside of a hospital setting.

Managing Anxiety, Stress, and Depression with Yoga

Yoga, a combination of breathing techniques, physical postures, and meditation, has been used successfully to reduce stress, lower blood pressure, and to improve concentration, sleep, and digestion, among other things. Several studies have shown yoga to effectively improve psychological symptoms and mental health. A recent meta-analysis of 10 studies, covering 762 cancer patients, concluded that yoga produced significant improvements in anxiety, depression, distress, and stress. Although relatively few studies of yoga have been conducted with cancer patients to date, the technique is clearly very promising.

Managing Anxiety, Stress, and Depression with Music Therapy

Music therapists connect with their patients through sound and song, rather than words. As musicians who are also trained as counselors, they typically bring portable instruments to the bedside, allowing patients to participate in playing, singing, or writing songs. This type of therapy often benefits both the patient and his or her family. It can reduce anxiety, depression, and pain, as well as encourage communication.

Other Things That May Help Manage Anxiety, Stress, and Depression

Acupuncture may also help to alleviate stress, anxiety, and depression, although this has not been thoroughly studied to date. In one high-quality trial, patients who had undergone surgery for various cancer diagnoses received both acupuncture and Swedish massage sessions on the first two days after their operations. This combination of complementary therapies produced a significant reduction in depression compared to patients who received usual care, as well as substantial reductions in pain scores.[7]

Acupuncture also has been shown to reduce anxiety prior to surgery, although it is not clear whether it has similar effects on general anxiety in cancer patients. A few studies suggest that it can enhance mood in breast and prostate cancer patients undergoing hormonal therapy (mood disturbance is a common side effect). Furthermore, many patients find acupuncture to be a relaxing and rewarding experience.

Many patients try various herbs and dietary supplements to reduce anxiety and depression. Saint-John's-wort is a notable example, because it may be as effective as placebo or standard antidepressants for mild-to-moderate depression. However, this herb can have significant interactions with many drugs and should not be used by patients on chemotherapy or other prescription medications. Similarly, another herb called kava kava was found to be effective for anxiety, stress, and insomnia, but it may cause liver damage. It is advisable to discuss any supplements you plan to take with your physician to ensure there won't be any harmful interactions.

Notes

1. Carlson LE, Speca M, Patel KD, Goodey E. Mindfulness-based stress reduction in relation to quality of life, mood, symptoms of stress, and immune parameters in breast and prostate cancer outpatients. *Psychosom Med.* 2003 Jul–Aug;65(4):571–81.

2. Piet J, Würtzen H, Zachariae R. The effect of mindfulness-based therapy on symptoms of anxiety and depression in adult cancer patients and survivors: A systematic review and meta-analysis. *J Consult Clin Psychol.* 2012 Dec;80(6):1007–20.

3. Devine EC, Westlake SK. The effects of psychoeducational care provided to adults with cancer: meta-analysis of 116 studies. *Oncol Nurs Forum.* 1995 Oct;22(9):1369–81.

4. Hernandez-Reif M, Ironson G, Field T, Hurley J, et al. Breast cancer patients have improved immune and neuroendocrine functions following massage therapy. *J Psychosom Res.* 2004 Jul;57(1):45–52.

5. Ahles TA, Tope DM, Pinkson B, Walch S, et al. Massage therapy for patients undergoing autologous bone marrow transplantation. *J Pain Symptom Manage.* 1999 Sep;18(3):157–63.

6. Grealish L, Lomasney A, Whiteman B. foot massage: a nursing intervention to modify the distressing symptoms of pain and nausea in patients hospitalized with cancer. *Cancer Nurs.* 2000 June;23(3):237–43.

7. Mehling WE, Jacobs B, Acree M, Wilson L, et al. Symptom management with massage and acupuncture in postoperative cancer patients: a randomized controlled trial. *J Pain Symptom Manage.* 2007 Mar;33(3):258–66.

Nausea and Vomiting

Most often associated with chemotherapy, nausea and vomiting are side effects that many cancer patients experience. This is not only an issue during treatment, as nausea can be "anticipatory," meaning it can start in advance of chemotherapy. The sight of the hospital might trigger nausea because of its association with chemotherapy in the mind of the patient. Sometimes delayed, low-grade nausea can also continue for a few days after treatment.

Fortunately, there are a variety of treatments that can help. Medicines called antiemetics are fairly effective at reducing nausea and vomiting symptoms and are the first line of defense. Several complementary therapies, such as acupuncture, mind-body, and massage, can have similar effects, or even extend the effects of drugs when used together. These complementary options can be used alone for mild nausea, and are often especially helpful for anticipatory nausea before chemotherapy or delayed nausea afterward. Antiemetic drugs are not always as helpful in these cases, and complementary therapies can help fill that void.

Managing Nausea and Vomiting with Acupuncture

Acupuncture is particularly effective as a complementary treatment for nausea and vomiting in cancer patients. It can help control these symptoms after chemotherapy, radiation, and surgery, and acupuncture's effects can last for hours if not longer. The most commonly studied acupuncture point for relief of such symptoms is called Neiguan or PC6. This point is centered on the wrist about two and a half finger widths up from the crease between hand and wrist. Several variations of acupuncture have been studied, including electroacupuncture, in which the needles are hooked up to a device that generates a slight electric current.

In one trial of breast cancer patients receiving a particularly nausea-inducing form of chemotherapy, electroacupuncture diminished symptoms of both nausea and vomiting. Compared to patients taking only antiemetic drugs, those who received electroacupuncture at the PC6 point once daily for 5 days had significantly fewer instances of vomiting. Patients in the acupuncture group had an average (median) of 5 episodes, compared to 15 in the medication-only group.[1]

Notably, the well-respected Cochrane Collaboration published reviews on this topic in 2006 and 2009. After examining all of the existing evidence, they concluded that acupuncture can reduce nausea and vomiting produced in cancer patients by chemotherapy or surgery. The first, published in 2006, evaluated 11 randomized controlled trials and determined that electroacupuncture helps reduce chemotherapy-induced nausea and vomiting. Further, they found that self-acupressure—in which the patient stimulates certain acupoints on their own by pressing, without needles—can help prevent nausea.[2]

The second Cochrane review, published in 2009, concluded that acupuncture at the PC6 acupoint on the wrist can effectively reduce nausea and vomiting after surgery. This was based on an examination of 40 prior randomized controlled trials. It was not clear, however, whether acupuncture was more effective than conventional antiemetic drugs alone (no significant difference was found).[3]

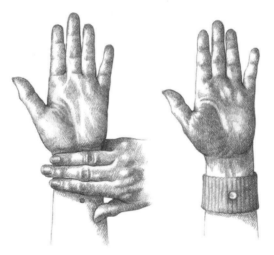

The P6 acupressure point can be located three fingers down from the crease of the wrist. Acupressure wristbands apply some pressure and must be precisely placed.

Remarkably, needles may not even be required to reduce nausea in this way. A recent randomized controlled trial in craniotomy patients found that transcutaneous electrode stimulation—that is, electrical stimulation without actually inserting a needle—at the PC6 acupoint before, during, and after surgery significantly reduced the incidence of nausea and vomiting over the course of 24 hours after the operation. Craniotomy is a procedure in which a section of bone is removed from the skull to expose the brain. Afterward, nausea and vomiting are very common, affecting up to 60 percent of patients despite the use of antiemetic medications. Patients who received the acupoint stimulation experienced a 40 percent lower incidence of nausea and a 60 percent decrease in vomiting compared to the placebo group, which received electrical stimulation at a non-acupoint.[4]

Although acupuncture is frequently more effective than usual care, some studies have found that some beneficial effects of properly performed acupuncture are mimicked by sham procedures, in which needles are inserted at non-acupoints (and should theoretically not have any effect). A recent investigation of acupuncture's effects on radiation-induced nausea, for example, found no significant difference in nausea frequency or intensity between the groups receiving true or sham acupuncture, although both groups experienced less intense nausea than patients receiving usual antiemetic care. As a result, some wonder whether acupuncture's benefits are at least partly the result of attention, doctor-patient interaction, or placebo response.[5]

Actually, it hardly matters exactly what produces the benefit—whether it is attention, doctor-patient interaction, placebo response, the acupuncture alone, a combination of these possibilities, or something else—so long as it works. Further research will help to sort this out, but for purposes of the patient, it hardly matters. Whatever the specific mechanism by which acupuncture works, it is very safe, relatively inexpensive, and can provide a significant benefit, particularly if nausea and related symptoms are an issue for you.

Managing Nausea and Vomiting with Mind-Body Therapies

Mind-body therapies, including meditation, hypnosis, and guided imagery, can greatly reduce symptoms such as nausea and vomiting. These methods help to relax and/or distract, and help put you in control of your body and mind.

Mind-body practices are particularly effective for *anticipatory* nausea, which is itself an example of the mind affecting the body. Just as vomiting can be a result of stage fright, there is no physical cause for anticipatory nausea. Rather, it is the body's response to the mind's anticipation of something unpleasant, such as chemotherapy. Using techniques such as self-hypnosis or guided imagery, you can learn to disrupt this process, to break the association and bring about relief.

Self-hypnosis was the one of the first mind-body techniques used to control nausea and vomiting. It puts you in a state of deep attention or "restful alertness" and makes you receptive to new ideas. Hypnosis has been shown to effectively treat anticipatory nausea in both adult and pediatric cancer patients. In a study of 54 pediatric patients, children were assigned to receive either hypnosis, distraction/relaxation techniques, or no intervention. Patients in the hypnosis group had a substantial reduction in both anticipatory and post-chemotherapy nausea. In contrast, nausea levels in the children who practiced distraction/relaxation remained unchanged, and symptoms in the no-intervention group consistently worsened over time. In another study, however, adding distraction and relaxation training reduced nausea prior to chemotherapy more effectively than when these techniques were not used.[6]

Training in guided imagery also can be valuable. This technique allows you to mentally remove yourself from your current situation and bring yourself to a place that is pleasant and relaxing. Without leaving the treatment room, you can imagine what you would be feeling, hearing, and seeing in this other, restful place. In so doing, it is possible to mentally block physical symptoms such as nausea and vomiting. Guided imagery is a relaxing technique that can be worthwhile for many aspects of day-to-day life, and it is not hard to learn.

Trained therapists can teach you self-hypnosis, guided imagery, or other mind-body techniques, and then you can continue to practice them on your own. Some hospitals may have these therapists on staff, otherwise, you can ask for a referral if you are interested.

Managing Nausea and Vomiting
with Massage Therapy

A few studies suggest that massage can help ease nausea in patients undergoing cancer therapy, most likely by providing a source of relaxation and distraction. In one small randomized controlled trial, 39 breast cancer patients currently undergoing chemotherapy were assigned to a massage group (five 20-minute visits with massage) or to a control group (five 20-minute visits, without massage). The massage treatments significantly reduced nausea levels. In another randomized study, patients' nausea scores decreased by about one-third after a single massage, with little or no change in the control subjects who did not receive the massage.

Massage therapy probably is most worthwhile if you have low-grade nausea, but it may not be the best or most helpful option if your nausea is more severe. Still, massage is extremely relaxing and can help treat a wide range of other symptoms, from pain to stress and anxiety.

Managing Nausea and Vomiting
with Music Therapy

Music therapy is conducted by specially trained professionals who use music to help alleviate symptoms. They bring portable instruments to the bedside and may perform music for or with patients. When used with typical antiemetic medications, music therapy may help to further reduce nausea and vomiting from chemotherapy. At the very least, it can relieve stress and reduce blood pressure, lower heart rate, and promote general well-being. Even something as simple as music can be very powerful.

Notes

1. Choo SP, Kong KH, Lim WT, Gao F, Chua K, Leong SS. Electroacupuncture for refractory acute emesis caused by chemotherapy. *J Altern Complement Med*. 2006 Dec;12(10):963–9.

2. PubMed Health. Acupuncture for nausea and vomiting which has been induced by having chemotherapy treatment. *Cochrane Database Syst Rev: Plain Lang Summaries*. First published: April 19, 2006.

3. PubMed Health. P6 acupoint stimulation prevents postoperative nausea and vomiting with few side effects. *Cochrane Database Syst Rev: Plain Lang Summaries*. First published: April 15, 2009.

4. Ni JW, Meng YN, Xiang HF, Ren QS, Wang JL. Effect of transcutaneous acupoint electrical stimulation on lipid peroxidation and cognitive function in patients experiencing craniotomy. PubMed. Zhen Ci Yan Jiu. 2009 Feb;34(1):52–6. Abstract in English; article in Chinese.

5. Azad A, John T. Do randomized acupuncture studies in patients with cancer need a sham acupuncture control arm? Correspondence. *J Clin Oncol*. 2013 June;31(16):2057–8.

6. Richardson J, Smith JE, McCall G, Pilkington K. Hypnosis for procedure-related pain and distress in pediatric cancer patients: a systematic review of effectiveness and methodology related to hypnosis interventions. *J Pain Symptom Manage*. 2006 Jan;31(1):70–84.

Hot Flashes

Hot flashes are a common side effect of treatment in people with hormone-dependent cancers, such as breast or prostate cancer. Hormone replacement therapy, which may be used to reduce hot flashes in postmenopausal women, cannot be used in breast cancer patients because it could stimulate growth of estrogen-sensitive tumors. Although some other drugs may help, they can have their own side effects. Many patients turn to complementary therapies, such as acupuncture or herb supplements, in hopes of finding safe and effective relief. Although much of the research on complementary therapies for hot flashes has been done with breast cancer patients, those results are likely applicable to prostate and other hormone-dependent cancers as well.

Managing Hot Flashes with Acupuncture

A growing body of evidence suggests that acupuncture may help to alleviate cancer treatment–related hot flashes. In one study, an analysis of 194 breast and prostate cancer patients found that hot flashes were reduced by about half in nearly 80 percent of the patients who received acupuncture. In a similar study, men who had received castration therapy for prostate cancer experienced a 70 percent reduction in number of hot flashes after 10 weeks of acupuncture.

In recent years, there have been an increasing number of high-quality randomized controlled trials of acupuncture for this symptom. One noteworthy study compared true acupuncture to sham acupuncture (essentially a placebo) in breast cancer patients who had previously undergone surgery and were currently taking tamoxifen. The trial found a significant reduction in hot flash frequency (both daytime and nighttime) in the true acupuncture group over 22 weeks. Moreover, a follow-up study further suggested that acupuncture may have had long-lasting benefits. In a questionnaire conducted two years later, several women stated that their hot flashes had remained "fewer and milder."

Another trial, however, found that true and sham acupuncture both reduced hot flashes, with no statistically significant difference between groups. Other studies have had similar effects, leading a few recent review articles to conclude that there is not yet sufficient evidence that acupuncture reduces hot flashes. In sham acupuncture, needles are usually inserted at non-acupoints, so it is possible that the simple act of inserting a needle may have beneficial effects. Alternatively, the observed benefits could be due at least in part to the interaction between acupuncturist and patient.[1]

Though it is not entirely clear how acupuncture works or what specific aspect of acupuncture treatment is effective, the fact remains that people who have acupuncture generally experience improvement in hot flashes. You may well find it helpful. Acupuncture is very safe when practiced by a trained provider, and most people find the experience enjoyable. Just be sure to find an acupuncturist who is trained and certified to work with cancer patients.

Managing Hot Flashes with Herbs and Other Dietary Supplements

Herbal remedies are often the first place people turn when looking for complementary remedies for hot flashes. Soy, red clover, flax seeds, a Chinese herb called Dong quai, yam, and evening primrose oil are among the commonly used botanical products. Each contains estrogen-like compounds (phyto-estrogens) that may mimic estrogen in the human body and thus ease symptoms of estrogen deprivation, such as hot flashes. Unfortunately, few studies have found these effective at providing relief. Moreover, there is some concern that they could exacerbate estrogen-sensitive cancers by promoting tumor growth, especially when taken in high doses. For a more detailed discussion of soy's risks and benefits, please see the diet chapter.

Studies of black cohosh (a popular herb) for treating hot flashes in breast cancer patients have had mixed results and have generally failed to prove that it reduces hot flashes any more than a placebo. However, black cohosh does not seem to have estrogenic activity. As such, it should not stimulate growth of hormone-sensitive tumors, as is a concern for certain other herbs.

Though not traditionally recommended for menopausal symptoms, vitamin E may benefit cancer patients suffering from hot flashes. A clinical trial found that 800 IU of vitamin E daily reduced hot flashes in breast cancer patients.[2] The effect was not that large, but vitamin E may be worth taking, especially because it is relatively safe and inexpensive. High doses of greater than 400 IU per day should not be taken for long periods of time or by patients with heart disease. Always make sure to discuss with your doctor before taking any herbs or supplements to be sure they are safe for your condition and that they won't interfere with your treatment.

As noted, herbs and other dietary supplements are biologically active products that may interfere with cancer treatment and reduce its ability to stop the cancer. It is essential not to take any herb or herbal compound during active cancer treatment. Memorial Sloan-Kettering Cancer Center (MSKCC) has developed a website and free app containing everything you need to know about herbs and other dietary supplements. Visit MSKCC.org/AboutHerbs for more information or to download the free app. Healthcare providers can also obtain additional information under the "Professionals" tab.

Notes

1. Rada G, Capurro D, Pantoja T, Corbalán J, et al. Non-hormonal interventions for hot flushes in women with a history of breast cancer. *Cochrane Database Syst Rev.* 2010 Sep 8:CD004923.
2. Barton DL, Loprinzi CL, Quella SK, Sloan JA, et al. Prospective evaluation of vitamin E for hot flashes in breast cancer survivors. *J Clin Oncol.* 1998 Feb;16(2):495–500.

Sexual Dysfunction

Sexual difficulties can be a side effect of treatment for certain kinds of cancer, including prostate, gynecologic, and breast tumors. Erectile dysfunction arising from surgical removal of the prostate or radiation therapy; pain and burning following surgery for gynecologic tumors; and impotence, pain, and other issues following hormonal treatment of breast and prostate cancer are common examples. Such side effects are difficult to contend with, but there are both conventional and complementary options that can help.

Treatment options depend on the specific kind of sexual symptoms, but counseling and medicines such as Viagra, for example, are often used. In the complementary realm, certain herbs and mind-body approaches, such as biofeedback and self-hypnosis, may be of significant value.

Managing Sexual Problems with Herbs and Dietary Supplements

A few botanical products may be of use for easing sexual side effects, although it is important to note that most studies have been not been conducted with cancer patients. Korean red ginseng, for example, has been studied in a few randomized controlled trials. In one, patients with erectile dysfunction reported a one-third improvement in sexual function after taking 900 milligrams of Korean red ginseng, with hardly any improvement in control subjects. Additionally, oral maca for men and both ArginMax (ginseng and ginko) and Zestra (a tropical plant product) for women have been shown to increase sexual desire. Because these supplements do not appear to act like hormones in the body, they should be safe for patients with hormone-sensitive tumors, such as breast or prostate cancer. Again, it is not clear to what degree these types of supplements are effective in cancer patients, although they may be worth trying. As always, be sure to discuss options with your doctor before taking any supplements.

Managing Sexual Problems with Mind-Body Therapies

Interventions that take advantage of the reciprocal relationship between mind and body, such as self-hypnosis and biofeedback, may help to relieve sexual dysfunction. Some data suggest that hypnosis may improve sexual function in men, though this research has not been conducted in patients with cancer-related sexual dysfunction. Particularly in cases where anxiety or depression is a contributing factor to sexual problems, it seems likely that various mind-body complementary approaches could help.

In another study, a combination of biofeedback therapy and pelvic floor exercise was found to effectively improve erectile dysfunction.

Managing Sexual Problems with Exercise

In a randomized trial of 55 men, some of whom had had their prostates removed, about half of whom were asked to perform daily pelvic floor exercises and to receive biofeedback guidance on lifestyle changes. The other half received only advice about lifestyle changes and served as controls. After three months, erectile function of men in the exercise and biofeedback group had improved significantly compared to those who received advice only. Moreover, even further improvement continued after six months.[1]

In general, physical activity may help to improve sexual function. In one study of prostate cancer patients who had received radiation therapy within the past 18 months, sexual function improved with increasing amounts of physical activity. That is, it appeared that the more men exercised, the greater the improvement.[2]

Notes

1. Prota C, Gomes CM, Ribeiro LH, de Bessa J Jr, et al. Early postoperative pelvic-floor biofeedback improves erectile function in men undergoing radical prostatectomy: a prospective, randomized, controlled trial. *Int J Impot Res*, Sep 2012;24(5).

2. Dahn JR, Penedo FJ, Molton I, Lopez L, Schneiderman N, Antoni MH. Physical activity and sexual functioning after radiotherapy for prostate cancer: beneficial effects for patients undergoing external beam radiotherapy. *Urology.* 2005 May;65(5):953–8.

Xerostomia

Xerostomia, or extreme dry mouth, is a common side effect among cancer patients who receive surgery and/or radiation therapy for head and neck cancer. The condition occurs when treatment damages the salivary glands. It can begin within a week of starting radiation treatment and can be a long-term problem. Besides being unpleasant, it can make eating and talking very difficult and contribute to dental issues such as cavities.

The good news is that new techniques for delivering radiation therapy are minimizing exposure and damage to the salivary glands. Available medication may provide some help in some cases, but has its own side effects. Perhaps the most encouraging development is that acupuncture appears to help resolve this condition. A growing body of evidence suggests that acupuncture safely improves xerostomia in many patients, including those for whom the medication does not work well and those who have suffered with this problem for many months and even years.

Managing Xerostomia with Acupuncture Treatment

Several studies suggest that acupuncture may improve radiation-induced xerostomia. In one case series, 50 patients received an average of five acupuncture treatments over the course of a month. Xerostomia was reduced by 10 percent or more in 70 percent of these patients, with about one-third of patients reporting improvements of 50 percent or more.

A small randomized trial of head and neck cancer patients who had previously undergone radiation therapy found that acupuncture led to significantly higher salivary flow and improved quality of life after 6 weeks, relative to patients who received sham acupuncture. Another study focused on patients who had undergone neck surgery for cancer at least three months prior. Weekly acupuncture treatments led to significant improvement in xerostomia compared to patients who had received usual care instead of acupuncture.

Perhaps most unique and promising was a recent high-quality randomized trial that demonstrated that acupuncture could help to minimize the effects of xerostomia when given prior to and on the same days as radiation treatment. This randomized trial compared the effectiveness of acupuncture versus usual care for preventing xerostomia in head and neck cancer patients (in this case, specifically patients with nasopharyngeal carcinoma). Acupuncture was administered three times per week for seven weeks, and a statistically significant improvement in xerostomia and quality of life was found starting the third week and persisting for six months, compared with patients who received usual care. Future trials with larger sample sizes hopefully will confirm these encouraging results.[1]

Moreover, brain imaging studies strongly suggest that acupuncture may be useful in treating xerostomia; one study found that acupuncture at a relevant acupoint produced a distinct brain activation pattern that was not observed with sham acupuncture, and that the pattern corresponded with an increase in salivary flow.[2]

Although a 2010 review article determined that there was not yet sufficient evidence to draw firm conclusions, it noted that the use of acupuncture for xerostomia is a promising area of research and worthy of further investigation.[3]

Because acupuncture is very safe, you might consider trying it if you have xerostomia. Again, be sure to use an acupuncturist who is trained to work with cancer patients.

Notes

1. Meng Z, Kay Garcia M, Hu C, Chiang J, et al. Sham-controlled, randomised, feasibility trial of acupuncture for prevention of radiation-induced xerostomia among patients with nasopharyngeal carcinoma. *Eur J Cancer*. 2012 Jul;48(11):1692–9.

2. Deng G, Hou BL, Holodny AI, Cassileth BR.. Functional magnetic resonance imaging (fMRI) changes and saliva production associated with acupuncture at LI-2 acupuncture point: a randomized controlled study. *BMC Complement Altern Med*, 2008 Jul 7;8:37.

3. O'Sullivan EM, Higginson IJ. Clinical effectiveness and safety of acupuncture in the treatment of irradiation-induced xerostomia in patients with head and neck cancer: a systematic review. *Acupunct Med*. 2010 Dec;28(4):191–9.

Insomnia and Sleep Disturbance

Many cancer patients face sleep problems, such as difficulty falling asleep, frequent nighttime waking, rising too early in the morning, or excessive sleeping during the day. Such symptoms may occur in more than 70 percent of people with cancer. Stress and anxiety about one's diagnosis, side effects of treatment, and many other factors can contribute. Moreover, poor sleep may contribute to other symptoms, such as fatigue or mood disturbances. Various medications for sleep work quickly and effectively, but they have their own side effects, including risk of dependence.

On the other hand, complementary approaches, such as relaxation or Tai Chi, take more time to learn but may lead to longer-term improvements in sleep quality. Research on complementary therapies for insomnia and other forms of sleep disturbance specifically in cancer patients is relatively limited. However, studies of sleep issues in the general population show that complementary therapies—particularly mind-body approaches—may be helpful, and these results are likely applicable to people with cancer.

Managing Sleep Problems with Mind-Body Therapies

Particularly because of the role that stress, anxiety, and other mental factors play in sleep issues, it is not surprising that complementary mind-body therapies may be of value. An analysis that pooled data from 59 studies, for example, found that psychological treatment averaging five hours of therapy meaningfully improved patients' ability to fall asleep faster and stay asleep longer. Moreover, the benefits lasted for at least six months. Other studies support those positive results. A National Institutes of Health consensus panel concluded that complementary techniques, particularly relaxation and biofeedback, improve some aspects of sleep. The magnitude of the improvements is somewhat less clear.[1]

Tai Chi, a slow-moving, meditative form of exercise, may also benefit those with trouble sleeping. In one small randomized trial of older adults with moderate sleep complaints, subjects received either 16 weeks of Tai Chi classes or a general health education program. Those who practiced Tai Chi experienced a significant increase in sleep quality compared to their counterparts who took health education. Specifically, measures of sleep quality, efficiency, and duration were improved.[2]

In general, mind-body therapies are an appealing approach for various cancer symptoms because they are inexpensive, can be used along with medicines or other conventional approaches, can be practiced on your own after initial training, have virtually no side effects, and are safe.

Managing Sleep Problems with Exercise

Besides helping to decrease fatigue, boost physical fitness, and even lower the risk of cancer recurrence, general physical activity has been shown to improve sleep. One clinical trial conducted in Taiwan found that an 8-week, home-based walking exercise program significantly improved sleep quality in cancer patients. Additionally, patients who exercised experienced reduced levels of pain and improved quality of life.

Another trial of breast and prostate cancer patients receiving radiation treatment had similar results. After taking part in a four-week, home-based exercise program, patients reported greater sleep improvements than did those who did not exercise. In a separate clinical trial of breast cancer patients receiving hormonal treatment, women who participated in a walking program 20 minutes per day, four days per week reported improved sleep quality within four weeks of starting the program.[3]

The list of favorable studies goes on and on. Given the well-known and evidence-based benefits of exercise for so many conditions, it's a no-brainer. Whether it's jogging, swimming, walking, or even gardening, you'll benefit from being as active as your condition allows.

Notes

1. http://consensus.nih.gov/1995/1995behaviorrelaxpaininsomniata 017html.htm

2. Irwin MR, Olmstead R, Motivala SJ. Improving sleep quality in older adults with moderate sleep complaints: a randomized controlled trial of Tai Chi Chih. Sleep. 2008 Jul;31(7):1001–8.

3. Rogers LQ, Hopkins-Price P, Vicari S, Markwell S, et al. Physical activity and health outcomes three months after completing a physical activity behavior change intervention: persistent and delayed effects. Cancer Epidemiol Biomarkers Prev. 2009 May.

Lymphedema

In breast cancer patients, lymphedema can occur as a troublesome complication of lymph node removal and/or after mastectomy. It involves chronic swelling of the arm due to the buildup of lymphatic fluid and affects about 30 percent of breast cancer survivors. Affected arms can become heavy, swollen, and thick, and the condition may lead to frequent infection. Fortunately, as surgery techniques become less invasive, the rates of developing lymphedema are lessening—though the risk remains.

In affected patients, intensive physical therapy is often required on a regular basis to reduce fluid buildup. Wearing tight stockings on the affected arm also is used in efforts to reduce swelling. The latest option is acupuncture, which is growing in acceptance and in pilot studies produced significant and enduring results, and may be a valuable tool for treating lymphedema. A major study is underway. Furthermore, early detection is key. Patients who begin treatment early, as soon as lymphedema begins, generally have the best results.

Managing Lymphedema with Massage Therapy

A program called complete decongestive therapy (CDT) is the most common therapy for lymphedema. It involves two phases: treatment and maintenance. The treatment phase generally involves physical therapy five days per week over the course of two to eight weeks as the girth and volume of the affected arm is reduced. The maintenance phase begins once these reductions have plateaued and continues for the long term with the goal of keeping the swelling down and preventing recurrence.

A specialized massage technique called manual lymphatic drainage (MLD) is a key component of the treatment phase. In MLD, the massage therapist uses a gentle pumping motion in order to mobilize lymph fluid trapped in the affected areas. One randomized trial that compared the effects of MLD with a simple lymphatic drainage technique found that MLD was significantly better. It reduced excess volume and skin thickness of the affected limb and also improved some quality-of-life measures.

Overall, complete decongestive therapy is effective—one large study of CDT found that it reduced arm volume by about 59 percent—but it is a long-term process. Unfortunately, lymphedema remains a distressing problem for many breast cancer patients. Emerging research suggests that acupuncture (see below) may be an important treatment option.

Managing Lymphedema with Acupuncture

Early clinical trials show that acupuncture can safely and effectively reduce limb swelling and other symptoms of lymphedema. As discussed throughout this chapter, acupuncture has been successfully studied to treat a wide range of conditions, including pain, hot flashes, chronic fatigue, nausea and vomiting, and xerostomia, and is found to be very safe.

In a recent pilot study conducted by our group at Memorial Sloan-Kettering Cancer Center, 33 women with breast cancer–related lymphedema received acupuncture treatment twice weekly for four weeks. The difference in circumference between each patient's affected and unaffected arms was used as a measure of the severity of lymphedema. One-third of the patients had a 30 percent or greater reduction in arm circumference difference after the four weeks of treatment, with no serious side effects reported.[1]

The effects of acupuncture treatment seem to last, making it potentially less time consuming, less expensive, and more effective, with much shorter periods of intervention required, than is the case for lymphedema massage treatment. Although these promising results will need to be confirmed in more rigorous, randomized trials, acupuncture may be worth considering if you have lymphedema that is not well managed by other treatment approaches.

Managing Lymphedema with Exercise

Despite past concerns that certain kinds of exercise could adversely affect cancer patients with lymphedema, physical activity has been shown not only to be safe but beneficial for lymphedema sufferers. Multiple studies show that physical activity such as upper body resistance training and/or vigorous aerobic exercise can actually reduce the incidence and severity of lymphedema.

One of these, a 2010 study by University of Pennsylvania researchers and published in the prestigious *Journal of the American Medical Association*, found that weight lifting in breast cancer patients at risk for lymphedema did not increase, and in fact decreased, its incidence. This randomized controlled trial involved 134 breast cancer survivors between one and five years after diagnosis who had had at least two lymph nodes removed but had not yet developed lymphedema. About half the women were assigned to a one-year weight lifting program, with 13 weeks of supervised instruction and then continuing on their own for the remaining nine months. The remainder of the women did not exercise. By the end of the year, 11 percent of the weight lifters developed lymphedema, compared to 17 percent of those who did not exercise.[2]

Given the many benefits of exercise, you need not let concerns about lymphedema stop you, and it very well may reduce swelling of your arm!

Notes

1. Cassileth BR, Van Zee KJ, Yeung KS, Coleton MI, et al. Acupuncture in the treatment of upper-limb lymphedema: results of a pilot study. *Cancer*. 2013 Jul 1;119(13)::2455–61.

2. Schmitz KH, Ahmed RL, Troxel AB, Cheville A, et al. Weight lifting for women at risk for breast cancer-related lymphedema: a randomized trial. *JAMA*. 2010 Dec 22;304(24):2699–705.

Neuropathy

Chemotherapy-induced peripheral neuropathy (CIPN) can be a painful symptom of certain chemotherapy regimens. It occurs in 10 to 20 percent of cancer patients who are treated with types of chemotherapy that are toxic to the nervous system, and usually involves pain, tingling, or other discomfort in the hands and/or feet. Treatment is sometimes stopped early in cases where this side effect becomes very severe. The symptoms sometimes resolve completely on their own after chemotherapy ends, but in many cases it remains a long-term problem. Certain drugs can help, but they come with their own side effects. Complementary therapies such as acupuncture, however, may be an effective option with fewer negative effects.

Managing Neuropathy with Acupuncture

It appears that acupuncture may ease chemotherapy-induced peripheral neuropathy, although this research is only in its early stages. Several promising pilot studies have been conducted. In one small study of 18 patients, 82 percent reported an improvement in symptoms after six weekly acupuncture sessions. In another, five out of six patients improved after 10 weeks of acupuncture, whereas only one of five improved among those who did not receive acupuncture. A slightly larger study involved 47 patients with peripheral neuropathy and objectively measured the degree of neuropathy by testing for changes in nerve conduction. Seventy-six percent of patients who received acupuncture improved, compared with only 15 percent of patients who received usual care but no specific treatment for neuropathy.[1]

These good results are not surprising, as acupuncture works through the nervous system and neuropathy is nerve damage or dysfunction. Collectively these studies are very encouraging. Given that acupuncture is very safe and that there are few other options for treating peripheral neuropathy, it is probably worth trying. High-quality clinical trials are in the works, and assuming they confirm these smaller studies, acupuncture may one day be a principal treatment option for chemotherapy-induced neuropathy.

Note

1. Schröder S, Liepert J, Remppis A, Greten JH. Acupuncture treatment improves nerve conduction in peripheral neuropathy. *Eur J Neurol*. 2007 Mar;14(3):276–81.

Appendix 1
Scam Alert

In the section that follows, we've listed several of the alternative approaches promoted to cancer patients that lack evidence to support their usage. Unproven approaches are dangerous to patients. Even when the therapy itself does not harm, people too often choose to shun conventional treatment and replace it with an alternative treatment that does nothing to diminish their disease.

All treatments listed here should be avoided.

Electrical Devices
Treatment type: Devices used to neutralize unhealthy energy of cancer cells

Also called: bioresonance therapy

Recommended: NO

Just the facts: Based on a belief that diseased tissues emit "electromagnetic oscillations" that are distinct from those of healthy cells. Devices promise to

diagnose and treat cancer and other diseases with
the use of electromagnetic fields and currents. Such a
claim is unsupported by science.

Energy Therapies

Treatment type: "Therapeutic touch" and application of
electromagnetic energy

Recommended: NO

Just the facts: Treatment applied on a belief that energy
fields exist around the body and that those fields can
be manipulated to treat disease and restore health.
Neither the existence of such energy fields nor the
ability to manipulate them for greater health is
supported by scientific evidence.

Entelev

Treatment type: Liquid

Also called: CanCell, Cantron, Protocel, and others

Recommended: NO

Just the facts: A brown liquid composed of several
chemical compounds, Entelev was created in 1936 by
chemist James Sheridan. Over the years, it has been
touted to treat a variety of chronic diseases in addition
to cancer, including HIV/AIDS, epilepsy, and
Alzheimer's disease. Animal studies have shown no
evidence of anticancer activity and the U.S. Food and
Drug Administration (FDA) made it illegal to

distribute across state lines in 1989.

Essiac

Treatment type: Herbal—available in a tea, pill, or liquid

Also called: Flor-Essence

Recommended: NO

Just the facts: This herb was originally popularized in the 1920s by a Canadian nurse named Rene Caisse. (In fact, the herb got its name from a reverse spelling of her name.) It started as a blend of four herbs, but other herbs have been added over the intervening years. While it is readily available online and in health food stores, there is lack of data on its safety and efficacy. No clinical evidence supports its use.

Healers

Treatment type: Touch

Also called: biofield therapy, healing touch, energy therapy

Recommended: NO

Just the facts: Therapeutic touch is practiced by passing hands above a patient's body to sweep away blockages in the patient's energy. Neither the existence of such energy fields nor the ability to manipulate them for greater health is supported by scientific evidence.

Homeopathic Medicine

Treatment type: Liquid

Recommended: NO

Just the facts: Begun in 1796 by Samuel Hahnemann, homeopathy is based on the theory that "like cures like." A substance that causes disease in a person can be used diluted to cure the same disease. Homeopathy has been the object of many clinical studies. At best, the homeopathic "medicines" had no better results than placebos, and at worst, homeopathy can be actively harmful.

Hyperbaric Oxygen Treatments

Treatment type: Patient placed in oxygen-rich chamber

Recommended: NO (has medical uses, but not in cancer treatment)

Just the facts: Although hyperbaric oxygen therapy is used to treat decompression sickness, carbon monoxide poisoning, and some types of burns, no scientific evidence supports its use in treating cancer.

Laetrile

Treatment type: Oral or intravenous

Also called: Amygdalin and "Vitamin 817"

Recommended: NO

Just the facts: Years of study found no anticancer activity.

Mind-Body Techniques

Treatment type: Meditation or biofeedback

Recommended: NO (can be used as complementary therapy with traditional treatment)

Just the facts: Based on the theory that patients can harness the power of their mind to heal their physical ills. Techniques, such as meditation and biofeedback, have been shown to reduce stress and promote relaxation and can be used as effective complementary therapies. However, claims that stress and other emotional issues can cause diseases such as cancer and correcting those issues alone can effectively treat those diseases have no support in scientific evidence.

Oxygen Therapy

Treatment type: Pills, intravenous oxygen, oral and intravenous hydrogen peroxide, and infusion of ozone-treated blood

Recommended: NO

Just the facts: There is no scientific evidence to support a tumor's need for an oxygen-poor environment, that oxygen is absorbed during digestion, or that any form of oxygen therapy has any efficacy. Even more concerning, serious adverse effects have been reported.

Prayer

Recommended: Not as an alternative treatment (can be used as complementary therapy with traditional treatment)

Just the facts: Although prayer may be helpful when used in conjunction with appropriate mainstream treatment, some patients elect to forego care in the hope that prayer alone will heal them. A recent research review found that, although certain individual studies suggest some benefit from intercessory prayer, there is no clear evidence that it has any impact on clinical outcomes. Prayer may be useful, but not as an alternative to mainstream cancer treatment.

Shark Cartilage

Treatment type: Powder and liquid

Recommended: NO

Just the facts: In the 1950s, surgeon John Prudden began testing the use of animal cartilage. It is purported to reduce the size of tumors by preventing blood vessel growth to the tumor. A few early animal studies supported an anti-tumor effect, but results from clinical studies since then have not been promising.

Appendix 2
Your Healthcare Team

Use this directory to record the name and contact information for all of your healthcare providers, including any complementary or integrative practitioners with whom you work. Having all of this information in one place can be invaluable.

Name	
Specialty	
Phone	
E-mail	
Address	

Visit www.sprypubcancer.com to download a printable sheet.

Name	
Specialty	
Phone	
E-mail	
Address	

Name	
Specialty	
Phone	
E-mail	
Address	

Name	
Specialty	
Phone	
E-mail	
Address	

Visit www.sprypubcancer.com to download a printable sheet.

Appendix 3
Sources of Survivor Information and Support

Included in this list are general cancer resources. Many, many resources exist for specific cancer types and specific patient needs—so many, in fact, that we could not attempt to list them all here.

Associations and Online Resources

American Cancer Society
  Cancer.org

American Society of Clinical Oncology (ASCO)
  cancer.net/publications-and-resources

American Institute for Cancer Research
  aicr.org

Cancer and Careers
  www.cancerandcareers.org

CancerCare
  800.813.4673 and cancercare.org

Cancer Financial Assistance Coalition
cancerfac.org

Cancer Support Community
888.793.9355 or cancersupportcommunity.org

Family Caregiver Alliance
800.445.8106 or caregiver.org

Federal Trade Commission (FTC) "Cure-ious? Ask."
Campaign to Avoid Cancer Scams
202.326.2222 or www.ftc.gov/bcp/edu/microsites/
curious/index.shtml

Food and Drug Administration (dietary supplement advice)
fda.gov/food/dietarysupplements/usingdietarysupple-
ments

Job Assistance Network
askjan.org

Journey Forward
journeyforward.org

Livestrong
855.220.7777 or livestrong.org

Memorial Sloan-Kettering Cancer Center AboutHerbs
website and smartphone app
mskcc.org/AboutHerbs.org

MyOncofertility.org
myoncofertility.org

National Cancer Institute
cancer.gov/cancertopics

National Cancer Institute, Office of Cancer Survivorship
dccps.nci.nih.gov/ocs/office-survivorship.html

National Cancer Survivors Day Foundation
ncsdf.org

National Center for Complementary and Alternative Medicine, Using Dietary Supplements Wisely
nccam.nih.gov/health/supplements/wiseuse.htm

National Coalition for Cancer Survivorship
888.650.9127 or canceradvocacy.org

National Institutes of Health Office of Dietary Supplements
ods.od.nih.gov

Patient Advocate Foundation
800.532.5274 (English) or 800.516.9256 (Spanish)
patientadvocate.org

Books

Cassileth BR. *The Alternative Medicine Handbook: The Complete Reference Guide to Alternative and Complementary Therapies.* New York: WW Norton, 1998. Japanese edition, 2000.

Bloch A, Cassileth BR, Holmes MD, Thompson CA (editors): *Eating Well, Staying Well during and after Cancer*. Atlanta, Georgia: American Cancer Society, 2004.

Cassileth BR, Deng G, Vickers A, Yeung KS. Integrative Oncology: *Complementary Therapies in Cancer Care*. Ontario, Canada: B.C. Decker, 2005. Korean editiom 2009.

Cassileth, BR. *The Complete Guide to Complementary Therapies in Cancer Care*. Singapore: World Scientific Publ Co, 2011. Chinese edition, 2013.

Mukherjee, S. *The Emperor of All Maladies: A Biography of Cancer*, Simon & Schuster, 2010.

Offit, P. *Do You Believe in Magic? The Sense and Nonsense of Alternative Medicine*, HarperCollins, 2013.

Abrams, D and Weil A. *Integrative Oncology*. Weil Integrative Medicine Library, Oxford University Press, 2009.

Markman M, Cohen L, Editors. *Integrative Oncology: Incorporating Complementary Medicine into Conventional Cancer Care* (Current Clinical Oncology). Humana Press, 2008.

American Cancer Society Complete Guide to Complementary & Alternative Cancer Therapies. American Cancer Society, 2009.

Glossary

Adapted from *The Complete Guide to Complementary Therapies in Cancer Care*, by Barrie Cassileth.

Acupoints Points or places along the body's meridians where needles or pressure are applied.

Acupressure Hand or finger pressure applied to an acupuncture point on the body.

Acupuncture Therapy using very thin needles inserted at designated points (acupoints) along meridians on the body to manage symptoms. In the context of traditional Chinese medicine, this is intended to balance the flow of energy and restore health.

Acute Having a short, sometimes severe course. Not chronic.

Alexander technique A type of movement therapy intended to reduce muscular tension. This technique is useful as a complementary therapy in treating stress, muscular fatigue, and neck and back pain.

Allopathic medicine Mainstream or modern medicine; based on principles proven through scientific research. Contrast with "alternative medicine."

Alternative medicine Therapies used in place of allopathic medicine; not proven by conventional scientific investigation.

Antioxidant A natural or synthetic substance, such as vitamin E, that prevents or delays the oxidation process in cells or tissue.

Aromatherapy The therapeutic use of scents distilled from plant oils; said to be useful in treating headaches, anxiety, and tension.

Art therapy The use of drawing, painting, and sculpting as therapy to treat behavioral or emotional problems; promotes self-expression.

Ayurvedic medicine An ancient traditional medicine system based on Hindu philosophy and ancient Indian civilization. The body is seen as a microcosm of the universe, consisting of the five elements of fire, water, earth, air, and ether. Each element corresponds to one of the five senses: sight, taste, smell, touch, and hearing. It embraces the concept of an energy force in the body similar to the Chinese concept of Qi, and emphasizes the balance of mind, body, and spirit to maintain health.

Bach flower remedies The use of oils from one or more of 38 different flowers to use as self-treatment for mental, emotional, and sometimes physical discomfort.

Benign Non-threatening to health or life; a noncancerous growth.

Biofeedback The use of electrical devices to recognize changes in body functions, such as heart rate, perspiration, and temperature, to achieve relaxation or muscle control. Sometimes used to treat incontinence and anxiety-related conditions.

Biopsy A diagnostic technique that examines tissues, fluids, or cells removed from the human body.

Botanical medicine Use of the entire plant or herb for therapeutic purposes.

Carbohydrate The major class of foods that includes starches, sugars, cellulose, and gums. Carbohydrates are a necessary part of the daily diet.

Carcinogen Any cancer-causing substance.

Cartilage Dense, flexible connective tissue found at the ends of some bones, in the nose, and elsewhere in the body.

Catheterization The process of inserting a catheter or small tube into a vessel, body cavity, or organ, such as the bladder or heart, in order to examine it with a tiny video camera, to inject or remove fluids, or to open passageways.

Chemotherapy The use of chemicals that do not harm most

normal tissue, but that attack fast-growing cells such as cancer cells.

Chi see Qi

Chiropractic The largest nonsurgical and drugless system of healing in the West. Chiropractic assumes that a smooth flow of nerve impulses from the brain to all parts of the body through the spinal column is necessary for maintaining homeostasis or equilibrium among different parts of the body, and thus good health. Misaligned vertebrae, called subluxations, are thought to interfere with the transmission of nerve impulses. The chiropractor uses manipulation to reposition spinal bones.

Chronic Continuing over a long period of time; not acute.

Complementary medicine Medical care that is adjunctive (used in addition to) mainstream medical care, also known as Integrative Medicine. Most complementary therapies are beneficial in promoting relaxation, reducing stress, and controlling symptoms.

Crystal healing Sometimes called gem therapy; uses quartz crystals and gemstones, which are believed to emit electromagnetic energy, for healing purposes; often used in combination with color therapy.

Cupping An ancient Chinese and Ayurvedic therapy that aims to lower blood pressure, improve circulation, and relieve muscle pain by making punctures in the skin and then covering them with a heated cup, which creates suction. Cupping was also used in colonial American medicine.

Dehydration The loss of water from the body. An abnormal and sometimes dangerous depletion of body fluids.

Energy therapies A broad range of treatments based on the use of various energy forms to heal illness and disease. Electroacupuncture, electromagnetic therapy, dental energy medicine, microwave energy, and other approaches use a variety of electrical devices. The transcutaneous electrical nerve stimulator (TENS) unit is useful for reduction of pain. The use of highly charged electric paddles in a hospital emergency department to restart a stopped heart is also a common practice. Most other uses are unproven.

Fasting Technically, abstention from eating. In alternative medicine, fasting is sometimes used to cleanse the body of impurities. This is based on a notion that when the body is not digesting food greater reserves of energy are available for use in immune function, cell growth, and elimination processes. Because the body is deprived of necessary energy resources during fasting, fasting can be dangerous.

Fat One of the three kinds of food energy, along with carbohydrates and protein. Fats are found in meat, poultry, fish, dairy products, and some vegetables. The U.S. food guide recommends only a small amount of fat from meat, poultry, and/or dairy products each day. Stored in the human body as adipose tissue, fat provides a major reserve source of energy. It also acts as "padding" between various organs of the body. It protects against cold and helps the body absorb certain vitamins. Excess dietary fat increases the risk of serious health problems.

Feldenkrais method A therapy designed to make the body work with gravity rather than against it by correcting physical habits of movement that put too much strain on muscles and joints.

Fiber Indigestible parts of plants, some soluble; others insoluble. In the human digestive system, fiber absorbs water and assists elimination. It is an essential part of a healthy diet.

Fungus A parasitic organism such as a mold or yeast that can infect the human body.

Gene A segment of a DNA molecule and the biological unit of heredity. It is self-reproducing and transmitted from parent to children.

Generic drug A medication without a specific brand name. After patent rights expire on brand-name medications, similar generic drugs are often produced and marketed at lower cost to the consumer.

Herb A plant or plant part valued for medicinal or other purposes. Culinary herbs are used as flavoring in cooking.

Herbal medicine Healing through the use of organic substances. One of the oldest forms of medical care, the ancient Egyptians, Chinese, Indians, and other early societies discovered that certain plants had curative properties. Myth and science over time have produced a system of therapies that range from the Doctrine of Signatures, in which an herb bearing physical characteristics similar to those of the illness would help cure, to the present-day pharmaceutical industry that produces medications synthesized from herbs. Chinese and Ayuravedic shamans, Indian medicine men, and modern practitioners have all used a wide variety of herbs to promote cures.

Homeopathy A system of medicine based on the concept of "like cures like" (the Law of Similars): symptoms are treated with extremely small amounts of drugs that would normally produce the same symptoms as the illness being treated. Homeopathy was developed by a German physician and chemist as an alternative to the more severe practices of bloodletting, vomiting, and other excesses of orthodox medicine practiced in the early 1800s.

Hormone One of many chemicals produced in the body by glands and certain organs. Hormones regulate activities of body systems, glands, organs and tissues, usually distant from their originating source. Hormones regulate blood sugar levels, women's menstrual cycles, and growth.

Hypnotherapy The use of hypnosis to treat or manage

certain medical and psychological problems; often used to treat stress, sleeping disorders, anxiety, fears and phobias, and depression; also used to assist smoking cessation and to overcome alcohol and substance abuse.

Infection The invasion of microorganisms and their subsequent multiplication in body tissues. A localized infection can go throughout the body if infecting microorganisms gain access to the lymphatic or vascular system.

Inflammation A protective response to injury or destruction of body tissue; a localized action to destroy or isolate injured tissue and the injurious agent.

Ligament A band of fibrous tissue that connects bones and cartilages and strengthens and supports joints.

Macrobiotics A system that emphasizes a life balance between yin and yang qualities. The diet is plant-based, comprised largely of whole grains, beans, soups (such as miso soup), and sea vegetables. It excludes meat and dairy, but fish is occasionally eaten.

Malignant Tending to metastasize and infiltrate. Used in describing cancerous tissue or tumors of potentially unlimited growth.

Mammography Low-dose X-rays of the breast to detect abnormalities such as cancer.

Meditation The process of focusing one's thoughts or

engaging in contemplation or reflection. As a complementary therapy, a method of reaching the mind's inner reservoir of creative thought and energy, as in Transcendental Meditation. Meditation can lower heart rate and address some blood pressure problems, help alleviate chronic pain, and reduce stress.

Meridians From traditional Chinese medicine, particularly acupuncture, the fourteen main channels of energy or life force that run up and down the body and head. Each meridian is said to affect a particular organ or body system.

Metabolism Collectively, all of the physical and chemical processes through which life is sustained. Metabolic processes are fueled by energy from nutrients in food.

Moxa Another name for dried mugwort. Used in moxibustion by burning on the ends of needles, or rolled into sticks or cones that are then heated. This is said to increase the flow of Qi in the body.

Moxibustion (or moxabustion) A therapy used by Chinese herbal practitioners. Mugwort is burned on or very close to the body at an identified affected site to increase circulation and promote healing.

Naturopathy (naturopathic medicine) A drugless therapy based on the body's own ability to heal itself, facilitated by a naturopathic physician trained to treat the cause rather than the effect of illness or disease. Treatments most often are diet and nutrition oriented with attention given to the patient's personal history and lifestyle.

Needling The primary action of acupuncture. Very thin needles are inserted into the skin at specific points along one of the many meridians, or life-force lines, on the body said to change the energy flow and thus promote healing.

Osteopathy A medical philosophy based on the concept that the body can fight disease if the body is in a "normal structural relationship, is adequately nourished, and is not adversely affected by environmental conditions." It follows accepted physical, surgical, and medicinal techniques for diagnosis and treatment. Some osteopathic physicians practice joint manipulation, postural re-education, and physical therapy to correct structural problems.

OTC (over the counter) Describes medications legally sold without a physician's prescription. Many cold remedies, aspirin, Tylenol, and products for indigestion are OTC medications.

Placebo effect Healing that results from the patient's belief in the treatment or the therapist.

Prana Ancient Indian concept of healing energy or "force," equivalent to traditional Chinese medicine's Qi.

Protein The primary and essential constituent of the protoplasm of all cells, consisting of complex combinations of amino acids. Protein, along with carbohydrates and fats, makes up the three primary dietary components. Meat, fish, poultry, eggs, and dried beans are major sources of protein.

Psychosomatic Concerned with the relationship between mind and body. Some bodily symptoms may be caused by mental or emotional disturbances; these are called psycho-somatic illnesses.

Qi According to ancient Chinese philosophy, Qi is the vital life "force" or energy that flows throughout the body along pathways that connect all organs and systems. Disruptions in the flow of Qi (pronounced "chee"; also spelled Chi) is said to cause imbalance and illness.

Qigong A traditional Chinese medicine regimen involving movements, breath regulation, and meditation, geared to balance Qi and maintain health.

RDA (Recommended Dietary, or Daily, Allowance) Guidelines developed by the Food and Nutrition Board of the U.S. National Research Council that set recommended levels of vitamins and minerals that are essential to good health.

Red blood cell Blood cells that contain the protein hemoglobin, which carries oxygen from the lungs to the body. A shortage of these cells causes anemia.

Reflexology A therapy that involves manipulation of the feet to promote balance among the body's systems.

Reflexologists believe that parts of the feet called "reflex points" are related to specific body organs or functions. Stimulation by finger and thumb massage is believed to eliminate energy blockages said to cause health problems.

Remission A condition during which symptoms of a disease are reduced.

Seasonal affective disorder (SAD) Depression associated with the dwindling sunlight that occurs in winter. Geographic location plays a major role: people living in northern areas are eight times more likely to experience SAD than are those living in more southern areas.

Sedative An agent or drug that calms or moderates nervousness or excitement.

Shiatsu means "finger pressure" in Japanese; an Asian bodywork or acupressure technique in which fingers at specific points apply a firm sequence of rhythmic pressure to "awaken" acupuncture meridians.

Soft tissues Tissues of the body other than bone or cartilage; includes organs, muscles, tendons, and ligaments.

Sound therapy An ancient method of healing based on the idea that everything in the universe, including the human body, is in a constant state of vibration and that even the slightest change in vibration can affect internal organs. It is believed that there is a natural frequency or note for each body part or organ, and that sound directed to a specific target can restore health to a body part whose vibration is off.

Swedish massage The most common form of massage, involving long gliding strokes, kneading, and friction on the superficial muscle layers; relieves muscle tension and promotes relaxation.

Symptom Evidence of disease; something that suggests the presence of a bodily disorder.

Syndrome A group of symptoms that occur together to produce a specific abnormality.

Systemic Relating to or affecting the body in general.

Tai Chi An ancient Chinese system of gentle exercise or precision movement and breathing that develops balance, control, and relaxation, and has calming effects. Tai Chi is used to treat stress-related problems and for rehabilitation after surgery, injury, and illness.

Tendon The fibrous cord attached to muscles and bones.

TENS (transcutaneous electrical nerve stimulation) An electric device often used to treat affected nerves to relieve pain; accepted in mainstream medicine as a useful treatment for some diagnoses involving pain associated with the nervous system.

Tincture An alcohol or alcohol-and-water solution prepared from a plant or medicine.

Toxin A poisonous substance produced by the metabolic activities of a living organism. Toxins usually are capable of inducing antibody formation in the body.

Traditional Chinese Medicine (TCM) A complex healing system based on thousands of years of practice in the healing arts.

Vein The vessel through which blood that is low in oxygen passes from various body parts or organs back to the heart.

Viruses Minute infectious agents capable of reproducing only in living host cells. Viral diseases include the common cold, influenza, mononucleosis, and AIDS.

Visualization A relaxation therapy based on the formation of meaningful images in the mind. Mental pictures are used to achieve relaxation, reduce heart rate, and heal illness.

Vitamins Organic substances in small quantities that are vital to nutrition and good health. Found in natural foods and sometimes produced by the body. They are identified by letters and letter-number combinations (such as A, B, B_2) and sometimes by their chemical names (such as niacin and pantothenic acid).

White blood cells The primary resource in the immune system and the body's defense mechanism against disease. White blood cells attach themselves to infectious microbes and usually produce antibodies to destroy invaders.

Yin/yang Complementary but opposing qualities assigned to everything in the natural world as part of ancient Chinese cosmology. Everything has a yin and a corresponding yang, as in night and day, hot and cold. The human body is said to have both yin and yang organs, which must produce a balance by operating in pairs. A balance of yin and yang forces in the body is assumed to create good health. Illness is thought to result when yin and yang are not balanced.

Yoga An ancient Eastern philosophy of health and well-being. It is also an exercise system that combines movement and simple poses with deep breathing and meditation to unite the human soul with a universal spirit. Prana, a life energy, is believed to flow through and vitalize the body. Those who practice yoga strive for a deep meditative state that promotes relaxation and reduces stress. It is a gentle exercise regimen suited to virtually any group. Yoga has been practiced as early as 3000 BC.

Index

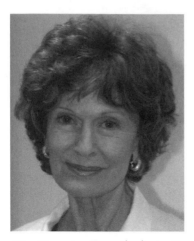

Barrie R. Cassileth, MS, PhD

Dr. Barrie Cassileth is Laurance S. Rockefeller Chair and
Chie emorial
Slo k City.
Sin lished
pro ; in In-
teg ership
car thera-
pie cludes
ex tbook
ch nilies.
Sh to the
U. native
M ry and
Al tional
an Cancer
So mmit-
tee nding
Pr